ADVANCES IN
Vascular Surgery

VOLUME 5

ADVANCES IN
Vascular Surgery

ADVANCES IN

Vascular Surgery

VOLUME 5

Editor-in-Chief
Anthony D. Whittemore, M.D.

Professor of Surgery, Harvard University Medical School; Chief, Division of Vascular Surgery, Brigham and Women's Hospital, Boston, Massachusetts

Associate Editors
Dennis F. Bandyk, M.D.

Professor of Surgery, University of South Florida College of Medicine; Director, Vascular Surgery Division, Tampa, Florida

Jack L. Cronenwett, M.D.

Professor of Surgery, Dartmouth Medical School; Chief, Section of Vascular Surgery, Dartmouth–Hitchcock Medical Center, Lebanon, New Hampshire

Norman R. Hertzer, M.D.

Chairman, Department of Vascular Surgery, Cleveland Clinic Foundation, Cleveland, Ohio

Rodney A. White, M.D.

Professor of Surgery, University of California at Los Angeles School of Medicine; Chief of Vascular Surgery, Associate Chairman, Department of Surgery, Harbor—University of California at Los Angeles Medical Center, Torrance, California

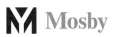 Mosby

St. Louis   Baltimore   Boston   Carlsbad   Chicago   Naples   New York   Philadelphia   Portland
London   Madrid   Mexico City   Singapore   Sydney   Tokyo   Toronto   Wiesbaden

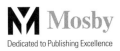

Dedicated to Publishing Excellence

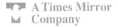
A Times Mirror
Company

Publisher: Cynthia Baudendistel
Acquisitions Editor: Gina G. Byrd
Developmental Editor: Susan Fox
Manuscript Editor: Amanda Maguire
Project Supervisor, Production: Joy Moore
Production Assistant: Laura Bayless
Illustrations and Permissions Coordinator: Chidi C. Ukabam

Printed in the United States of America
Composition by The Clarinda Company
Printing/binding by The Maple-Vail Book Manufacturing Company

Mosby–Year Book, Inc.
11830 Westline Industrial Drive
St. Louis, Missouri 63146

International Standard Serial Number: 1069–7292
International Standard Book Number: 0–8151–9409–9

Contributors

Dennis F. Bandyk, M.D.
Professor of Surgery; Director, Division of Vascular Surgery; The University of South Florida College of Medicine, Division of Vascular Surgery, Tampa, Florida

Keith D. Calligaro, M.D.
Section of Vascular Surgery, Pennsylvania Hospital/University of Pennsylvania School of Medicine, Philadelphia, Pennsylvania

Richard P. Cambria, M.D.
Associate Professor of Surgery, Harvard Medical School, Boston, Massachusetts; Visiting Surgeon, Department of Vascular Surgery, Massachusetts General Hospital, Boston, Massachusetts

Michael D. Dake, M.D.
Chief, Department of Cardiovascular and Interventional Radiology, Assistant Professor, Department of Cardiovascular and Interventional Radiology, Stanford University Hospital, Stanford, California

Rahul Dandura
Section of Vascular Surgery, Pennsylvania Hospital/University of Pennsylvania School of Medicine, Philadelphia, Pennsylvania

J. Kenneth Davison, D.D.S., M.D.
Associate Professor of Anesthesia, Harvard Medical School, Boston Massachusetts; Anesthetist, Department of Anesthesia, Massachusetts General Hospital, Boston, Massachusetts

Dominic A. DeLaurentis, M.D.
Section of Vascular Surgery, Pennsylvania Hospital/University of Pennsylvania School of Medicine, Philadelphia, Pennsylvania

Edward B. Diethrich, M.D.
Medical Director, Arizona Heart Institute, Phoenix, Arizona; Chief of Cardiovascular Surgery and Chairman of the Department of Cardiovascular Services, Columbia Medical Center-Phoenix, Phoenix, Arizona

Yves-Marie Dion, M.D., M.Sc., F.A.C.S., F.R.C.S.C.
Associate Professor of Surgery, Centre Hospitalier Universitaire de Québec, Pavillon St-François d'Assise, Université Laval, Québec, Québec, Canada

Matthew J. Dougherty, M.D.
Section of Vascular Surgery, Pennsylvania Hospital/University of
Pennsylvania School of Medicine, Philadelphia, Pennsylvania

Mark F. Fillinger, M.D.
Assistant Professor of Surgery, Section of Vascular Surgery,
Dartmouth-Hitchcock Medical Center, Lebanon, New Hampshire

Carlos R. Gracia, M.D., F.A.C.S.
Director, California Laparoscopic Institute, San Ramon Regional Medical
Center, San Ramon, California

John W. Hallett, Jr., M.D.
Professor of Surgery, Mayo Clinic, Rochester, Minnesota

Jeffrey L. Kaufman, M.D.
Division of Vascular Surgery, Baystate Medical Center, Springfield,
Massachusetts

Stephen T. Kee, M.B., F.R.C.R.
Assistant Professor, Department of Cardiovascular and Interventional
Radiology, Stanford University Hospital, Stanford, California

Timothy K. Liem, M.D.
Vascular Surgery Resident Physician, Department of Surgery, University
of Missouri–Columbia, Columbia, Missouri

William C. Mackey, M.D.
Associate Professor of Surgery, Tufts University School of Medicine,
Boston, Massachusetts; Chief, Vascular Surgery, New England Medical
Center Hospitals, Boston, Massachusetts

Mark R. Nehler, M.D.
Fellow, Department of Surgery, Division of Vascular Surgery, Oregon
Health Sciences University, Portland, Oregon

John M. Porter, M.D.
Professor of Surgery, Department of Surgery, Division of Vascular
Surgery, Oregon Health Sciences University, Portland, Oregon

Carol A. Raviola, M.D.
Section of Vascular Surgery, Pennsylvania Hospital/University of
Pennsylvania School of Medicine, Philadelphia, Pennsylvania

Robert Y. Rhee, M.D.
Assistant Professor of Surgery, Section of Vascular Surgery, Department
of Surgery, University of Pittsburgh School of Medicine, Pittsburgh,
Pennsylvania

Charles P. Semba, M.D.

Associate Professor, Department of Cardiovascular and Interventional Radiology, Assistant Professor, Department of Cardiovascular and Interventional Radiology, Stanford University Hospital, Stanford, California

Donald Silver, M.D.

W. Alton Jones Distinguished Professor and Chairman, Department of Surgery, University of Missouri–Columbia, Columbia, Missouri

David L. Steed, M.D.

Professor of Surgery and Director, Wound Healing Clinic, Section of Vascular Surgery, Department of Surgery, University of Pittsburgh School of Medicine, Pittsburgh, Pennsylvania

Lloyd M. Taylor, Jr., M.D.

Professor of Surgery, Department of Surgery, Division of Vascular Surgery, Oregon Health Sciences University, Portland, Oregon

Marshall W. Webster, M.D.

Professor of Surgery and Chief, Section of Vascular Surgery, Department of Surgery, University of Pittsburgh School of Medicine, Pittsburgh, Pennsylvania

W. Kent Williamson, M.D.

Resident, Department of Surgery, Division of Vascular Surgery, Oregon Health Sciences University, Portland, Oregon

R. Eugene Zierler, M.D.

Professor of Surgery, Department of Surgery, Division of Vascular Surgery, University of Washington School of Medicine, Seattle, Washington

Contents

PART V Aortic Disease

Critical Pathways for Abdominal Aortic Aneurysms.
By Keith D. Calligaro, Rahul Dandura, Matthew J. Dougherty, Carol A. Raviola, and Dominic A. DeLaurentis

Epidural Cooling for the Prevention of Spinal Cord Ischemic Complications After Thoracoabdominal Aortic Surgery.
By Richard P. Cambria and J. Kenneth Davison

Utility of Spiral CT in the Preoperative Evaluation of Patients with Abdominal Aortic Aneurysms.
By Mark F. Fillinger

The Role of Growth Factors in Lower Extremity Ischemia and Nonhealing Wounds.

By Robert Y. Rhee, Marshall W. Webster, and David L. Steed

PART I

Carotid Artery Disease

CHAPTER 1

Surgical Management of Recurrent Carotid Stenosis

William C. Mackey, M.D.
Associate Professor of Surgery, Tufts University School of Medicine, Boston, Massachusetts; Chief, Vascular Surgery, New England Medical Center Hospitals, Boston, Massachusetts

S ignificant (50% or greater) recurrent carotid stenosis occurs in 7% to 22% of the patients who have undergone carotid endarterectomy.[1–4] The results of postendarterectomy surveillance with duplex US at Tufts University–New England Medical Center are presented in Table 1. As indicated, 50% or greater restenosis or carotid occlusion has developed in approximately 16% of our patients at some time during a mean follow-up period of nearly 53 months.[1]

Recurrent stenosis may occur at any postendarterectomy interval. Lesions detected within the first several months after endarterectomy are likely to represent residual stenosis rather than re-

TABLE 1.
Recurrent Carotid Stenosis Detected by Duplex Ultrasonography During a Mean Follow-up Interval of 53 Months

Normal	205/348	58.9%
30%–49% restenosis	87/348	25.0%
50%–74% restenosis	26/348	7.5%
75%–99% restenosis	19/348	5.5%
Occlusion	11/348	3.2%

(Courtesy of Mackey WC, Belkin M, Sindhi R, et al: Routine post-endarterectomy duplex surveillance: Does it prevent late stroke? *J Vasc Surg* 16:934–940, 1992.)

Advances in Vascular Surgery®, vol. 5
©1997, Mosby–Year Book, Inc.

1

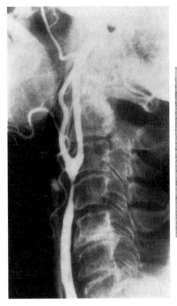
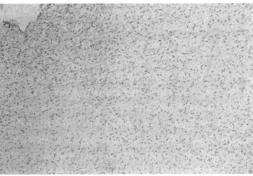

FIGURE 1.

Arteriographic and histologic appearances of early (less than 24 months) recurrent stenosis related to neointimal fibrous hyperplasia.

current disease. True restenoses occurring within 24 months of the original operation are invariably related to neointimal fibrous hyperplasia, whereas those occurring later than 36 months after the initial endarterectomy usually represent either atherosclerotic degeneration of a hyperplastic lesion or true recurrent atherosclerosis.[5, 6] Figure 1 illustrates the smooth, tapered arteriographic appearance and the homogeneous fibrous histologic characteristics typical of early restenosis. In comparison, Figure 2 demonstrates the irregular arteriographic appearance and the atherosclerotic histology of late restenosis.

Risk factors for recurrent stenosis include hyperlipidemia, hypertension, and tobacco use. Female sex, noted in some studies to be associated with an increased risk for recurrence, may not be an independent risk factor. Minor technical defects that were not corrected at the initial operation are probably less important than systemic factors in determining the risk of significant restenosis.[7] Therefore, risk factor modification may be an effective means of decreasing the incidence of restenosis. The liberal use of patch closure during the primary endarterectomy may reduce the incidence of significant recurrence, but there has been no convincing demonstration that patching improves short- or long-term clinical outcome.

The natural history of untreated recurrent carotid stenosis has not been described in detail, but despite the frequency with which significant recurrence is detected, transient ischemic attacks (TIAs) or strokes related to recurrent stenosis are unusual. The clinical outcome for 55 patients with 50% or greater recurrent carotid stenosis at New England Medical Center is presented in Table 2. More than half of our patients with significant restenosis remained asymptomatic without intervention and did not progress to carotid occlusion during a mean follow-up of 53 months.[1] Of interest, however, is the fact that there were 2 unheralded strokes related to sudden carotid occlusion in this group, as well as another 8 carotid occlusions that did not result in permanent neurologic deficits. Consequently, 10 (18%) of our 55 patients with uncorrected restenosis of 50% or greater experienced an adverse outcome.

Using our carotid follow-up registry, we evaluated all patients who sustained strokes more than 30 days after carotid endarterectomy.[8] Thirty-five (5.1%) of the 688 patients in this registry have had subsequent strokes. Eleven (31%) of these 35 strokes were clearly related to recurrent stenosis. Only 3 (15%) of the 20 strokes occurring within 36 months of endarterectomy were related to recurrent stenosis, however, compared with 8 (53%) of 15 strokes oc-

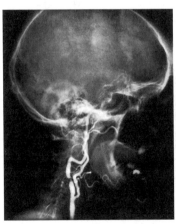
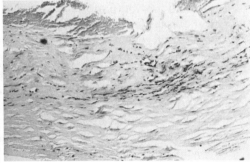

FIGURE 2.

Arteriographic and histologic appearances of late (greater than 36 months) restenosis related to recurrent atherosclerosis.

TABLE 2.

Available Clinical Outcome in Patients With Recurrent
Carotid Stenosis

Asymptomatic, no occlusion, no reoperation	29/55	52.8%
Occlusion with no neurologic events	8/55	14.5%
Reoperation for transient ischemia	8/55	14.5%
Reoperation for asymptomatic restenosis	8/55	14.5%
Unheralded stroke	2/55	3.6%

(Courtesy of Mackey WC, Belkin M, Sindhi R, et al: Routine post-endarterectomy duplex surveillance: Does it prevent late stroke? *J Vasc Surg* 16:934–940, 1992.)

curring after 36 months. Accordingly, early restenosis associated with neointimal fibrous hyperplasia appears less likely to result in stroke than does later restenosis related to atherosclerotic degeneration of the previous endarterectomy site. Similarly, Carballo et al.[9] found that no neurologic events occurred in 22 patients who were discovered to have early recurrent stenosis (50% to 75%) less than 12 months after their original carotid procedures. Five of these 22 patients underwent reoperations for critical asymptomatic recurrent stenosis, whereas the remaining 17 remained under nonoperative surveillance. In comparison, 26 other patients in the same series had late (greater than 12 months) restenosis; 3 (12%) of these lesions progressed to occlusion with 2 major strokes, and another 4 patients (15%) had related TIAs. None of the 26 patients with late recurrent lesions had greater than 75% restenosis at the time of their initial detection, and for this reason, no elective reoperations were performed. In aggregate, 7 (27%) of these 26 patients experienced TIAs, strokes, and/or carotid occlusion, whereas none of the 17 patients with early 50% to 75% restenosis had unfavorable outcomes.

Neointimal hyperplastic lesions have a smooth, fibrous consistency, whereas recurrent atherosclerotic lesions are more likely to have irregular, ulcerated surfaces lined by thrombus and pultaceous debris (see Figs 1 and 2). These important differences in plaque morphology may explain the observed differences in clinical behavior that are now known to be related to early and late recurrences.[10]

INDICATIONS FOR REOPERATION

Because stroke related to recurrent stenosis is uncommon and reoperative carotid surgery generally has higher complication rates than do primary procedures, the indications for "redo" carotid end-arterectomy should be relatively strict. Most neurologists and vascular surgeons agree that patients who have symptoms that are related to severe recurrent stenosis should undergo reoperations, although no compelling data exist to substantiate this approach. The role of "redo" endarterectomy is even less certain in the management of asymptomatic recurrences. Irrespective of whether patients with recurrent carotid stenosis are symptomatic or asymptomatic, however, their indications for elective surgical treatment may not be equivalent to those for primary intervention because of their higher risk for cranial nerve injuries and the perception that the natural history of untreated recurrent lesions may be different from that for primary carotid disease. "Redo" carotid endarterectomy is appropriate only if the surgical risk is low and the long-term outcome for patients who are subjected to reoperation is better than that for similar patients who are managed nonoperatively.

In our most recent series of 48 "redo" carotid endarterectomies, there was 1 operative mortality (2.1%) related to myocardial ischemia and 1 stroke (2.1%).[11] Thus, we have documented that reoperations can be performed with sufficient safety at our own center to be potentially effective in reducing morbidity from recurrent stenosis. As indicated earlier, the natural history of recurrent stenosis is not necessarily benign, with an adverse outcome (stroke and/or carotid occlusion) in 10 (18%) of our 55 patients with 50% or greater restenosis monitored by duplex scanning. More recently, we have monitored another cohort of 40 asymptomatic patients with 50% or greater restenosis without intervention because of their advanced age, medical co-morbidities, or the fact that their disease did not appear to be severe enough to justify elective reoperations.[11] At a mean postoperative interval of 63 months, there was only 1 TIA (4.7%) and no strokes among 21 of these patients who had recurrent 50% to 75% stenosis. In comparison, the neurologic event rate was 33% (2 strokes and 1 TIA) for 9 other patients who had 70% to 99% stenosis, and strokes had also occurred in 3 of the 10 patients whose recurrent lesions had already progressed to occlusion by the time they were detected. The incidence of events in this series seemed to be more closely related to the degree of stenosis than to the timing ("early" vs. "late") of the recurrent lesion. These findings are unlike those of Carballo et al.[9] As already mentioned, early restenosis of moderate severity (50% to 75%) was associated with a benign course in their series, whereas late, moderate restenosis progressed to occlusion in 3 (12%) of 26 patients (with 2 major strokes) and caused TIAs in an additional 4 patients (15%).

TABLE 3.

Treatment Algorithm for Patients With Recurrent Carotid Stenosis

	Symptomatic		Asymptomatic	
Restenosis	**50%–75%**	**75%–99%**	**50%–75%**	**75%–99%**
Early (<24 mo)	?*	Reop	Monitor	Reop
Late (>24 mo)	Reop	Reop	?†	Reop

*A trial of medical management is usually appropriate in this group, surgery being reserved for failure of medical management or disease progression.
†Plaque morphology and patient co-morbidities should be carefully considered in this group.

Although critical (greater than 75%) asymptomatic restenosis is probably best treated surgically, the indications for reoperation in asymptomatic patients with only moderate restenosis are less clear and may depend more on the type of recurrent stenosis and its plaque morphology. Because they appear to have a rather benign natural history, we are somewhat more conservative in the management of early (24 month) lesions; only 27% of our reoperations have been performed within 2 years of the initial procedure, and these early reoperations were limited to patients with symptoms, greater than 90% restenosis, or both.[11]

Our current management strategy is summarized in Table 3. Reoperations are offered to all patients with critical restenosis unless age or co-morbid conditions preclude intervention. Asymptomatic patients with early 50% to 75% restenosis are monitored by serial duplex studies. Symptomatic patients with early 50% to 75% restenosis are thoroughly evaluated for other potential sources of their symptoms. These patients then may be treated medically, with reoperation reserved for failure of medical therapy or progression of their recurrent disease. Asymptomatic patients with late 50% to 75% restenoses must be evaluated on an individual basis. Those who have ominous plaque morphology (i.e., gross irregularity or ulceration) and acceptable surgical risk may be candidates for reoperation, whereas others may be treated medically and monitored by serial duplex studies.

SURGICAL TECHNIQUE

Meticulous dissection of the artery with adequate proximal and distal exposure is essential for the safe conduct of "redo" endarterectomy. Cranial nerve injury is the most frequent complication of reoperations and has been reported in about 15% of the cases.[11, 12] The frequency and potential morbidity of this complication underscore the importance of painstaking care in the initial arterial exposure. Ideally, the proximal and distal exposure should extend beyond the area of the primary operation, and it may be appropriate to maintain dissection outside the scar from the prior operation until proximal and distal control is attained to lessen the likelihood of embolization from arterial manipulation. This approach may be especially important in patients having friable, ulcerated lesions in conjunction with late recurrent stenosis. Mandibular subluxation may also be an appropriate adjunct in patients for whom very high exposure of the distal internal carotid artery is necessary.

The rationale for cerebral monitoring and protection techniques is no different for reoperations than for primary endarterectomy. Both routine shunting and selective shunting based on electroencephalography or internal carotid stump pressure are acceptable alternatives in "redo" endarterectomy. Because of the technical difficulty of many reoperations, however, regional anesthesia with neurologic monitoring in awake patients is often not applicable.

Endarterectomy may be very difficult in patients with early recurrent stenosis that is caused by neointimal fibrous hyperplasia. Persistent attempts to achieve an endarterectomy plane where none exists can result in disruption of the artery and the necessity for vein graft interposition. Nevertheless, the hyperplastic lesion can usually be shaved from the underlying arterial wall by using a fine blade and gentle blunt technique. Once an adequate flow surface has been obtained, either a patch of saphenous vein harvested from the thigh or a synthetic patch should be used to enlarge the luminal diameter in an effort to prevent a secondary recurrence. Reconstruction with a saphenous vein graft is also an acceptable option if a reasonable flow surface cannot be achieved.

Late recurrent stenosis related to atherosclerotic degeneration is usually amenable to standard endarterectomy. In this setting, an appropriate endarterectomy plane is often achieved without difficulty. Again, patch closure is almost always performed unless the artery is quite large and the recurrent lesion is confined to the common carotid artery and the proximal carotid bulb.

RESULTS

Using our stated criteria for patient selection and these guidelines for surgical technique, we have reported satisfactory results in patients requiring reoperations.[11, 12] Our perioperative stroke and mortality rate is 2.1% each. Transient postoperative cranial nerve palsies have occurred in 19% of our patients. Actuarial stroke-free rates have been acceptable (92% at 1 year and 83% at 5 years) and are only slightly less favorable than those after primary operations (97% at 1 year and 91% at 5 years).[11, 12] Furthermore, there were no significant differences in stroke-free rates from the time of the primary operation between our patients who required "redo" endarterectomy and those who did not.[12]

Because the incidence of stroke related to recurrent stenosis is so low, it is difficult to conclusively prove that reoperations further reduce stroke risk. Nevertheless, our data indicate that selected patients who have recurrent stenosis that is associated with some of the features (symptoms or severity) suggesting a risk for related stroke can be managed surgically with acceptable perioperative complication rates and with a long-term outcome similar to that for primary carotid procedures.[12] Careful patient selection and performance of the reoperation at a center with sufficient experience in reoperative carotid surgery are necessary to ensure that the potential benefit exceeds the operative risk in these patients.

REFERENCES

1. Mackey WC, Belkin M, Sindhi R, et al: Routine post-endarterectomy duplex surveillance: Does it prevent late stroke? *J Vasc Surg* 16:934–940, 1992.
2. Cook JM, Thompson BW, Barnes RW: Is routine duplex examination after carotid endarterectomy justified? *J Vasc Surg* 12:334–339, 1990.
3. Gelabert HA, El Massry S, Moore WS: Carotid endarterectomy with primary closure does not adversely affect the rate of recurrent stenosis. *Arch Surg* 129:648–654, 1994.
4. Nichols SC, Phillips DJ, Bergelin RO, et al: Carotid endarterectomy: Relationship of outcome to early restenosis. *J Vasc Surg* 2:375–381, 1985.
5. Stoney RJ, String ST: Recurrent carotid stenosis. *Surgery* 80:705–710, 1976.
6. Clagett GP, Robinowitz M, Youkey JR, et al: Morphogenesis and clinicopathologic characteristics of recurrent carotid disease. *J Vasc Surg* 3:310–323, 1986.
7. Reilly LM, Okuhn SP, Rapp JH, et al: Recurrent carotid stenosis: A consequence of local or systemic factors? The influence of unrepaired technical defects. *J Vasc Surg* 11:448–460, 1990.
8. Washburn WK, Mackey WC, Belkin M, et al: Late stroke after carotid endarterectomy: The role of recurrent stenosis. *J Vasc Surg* 15:1032–1037, 1992.

9. Carballo RE, Towne JB, Seabrook GR, et al: An outcome analysis of carotid endarterectomy: The incidence and natural history of recurrent stenosis. *J Vasc Surg* 23:749–754, 1996.

10. O'Donnell TF, Callow AD, Scott G, et al: Ultrasound characteristics of recurrent carotid disease: Hypothesis explaining the low incidence of symptomatic recurrence. *J Vasc Surg 2:26–41, 1985.*

11. O'Donnell TF, Rodriguez A, Fortunato J, et al: The management of recurrent carotid stenosis: Should asymptomatic lesions be treated surgically? *J Vasc Surg* 24:207–212, 1996.

12. Nitzberg RS, Mackey WC, Prendiville E, et al: Long-term follow-up of patients operated on for recurrent carotid stenosis. *J Vasc Surg* 13:121–127, 1991.

PART II

Brachiocephalic Disease

CHAPTER 2

Endovascular Treatment of Brachiocephalic Lesions With Angioplasty and Stents

Edward B. Diethrich, M.D.

Medical Director, Arizona Heart Institute, Phoenix, Arizona; Chief of Cardiovascular Surgery and Chairman of the Department of Cardiovascular Services, Columbia Medical Center-Phoenix, Phoenix, Arizona

The brachiocephalic vessels supply our most precious tissue, and occlusion of these vital channels may result in catastrophic consequences. In the United States, stroke is the third leading cause of death, with approximately a half million new strokes occurring each year. Stroke is also a significant cause of disability, and the cost of medical management for its victims is estimated to be as much as $20 billion per year.[1] Whereas the medical community takes careful aim at vascular disease with comprehensive preventive programs, vascular interventionists continue to perfect treatment regimens for those who already have occlusive disease. The intent of all cerebrovascular intervention is the prevention of stroke and alleviation of symptoms, and percutaneous transluminal angioplasty (PTA) and stenting are promising therapeutic entities.

In the coronary and peripheral vessels, angioplasty and stents have revolutionized the treatment of occlusive disease. Percutaneous transluminal angioplasty was first used in the brachiocephalic vessels to treat proximal aortic arch vessel lesions[2] and later to correct postsurgical stenosis in the common carotid artery.[3] Clearly, brachiocephalic angioplasty offers a number of advantages over surgical intervention: the incision (if needed at all) is insignificant, the duration of induced occlusion is very short, surgically inaccessible lesions are amenable to treatment, general anesthesia is not required, and the hospitalization period and need for postoperative surveillance may be reduced.

The application of PTA in the brachiocephalic vessels has met with controversy because of concern over the potential for thromboembolic complications. The safety and efficacy of this application, however, have been demonstrated, and angioplasty is now in routine use for lesions involving all the aortic arch branches. Technology is now taking us beyond angioplasty with the introduction and proliferation of devices that complement the already impressive results seen with percutaneous intervention. Stents are proving to be one of the most exciting interventional technologies ever; they have had a significant impact on the outcome of endoluminal treatment and have expanded therapeutic options in the arteries and veins. Stenting has been used with great success to improve luminal diameter and restore flow in occluded arteries, and results have quickly eclipsed those seen with laser and atherectomy procedures. The use of stents in proximal brachiocephalic lesions has enjoyed a good deal of success.[4–8]

A review of the techniques, technology, and clinical experience with brachiocephalic angioplasty and stenting is provided. Topics of discussion include anesthesia, access, imaging, management of complications, and a review of clinical results.

TECHNIQUES AND TECHNOLOGY

The use of new techniques and technologies in percutaneous intervention is revolutionizing therapeutic alternatives in the treatment of vascular occlusive disease. Experience at the Arizona Heart Institute indicates that a number of strategies may be successfully used in angioplasty and stenting procedures in the brachiocephalic vessels.

ANESTHESIA

The choice of anesthesia during percutaneous intervention is an important one. Although we have used general anesthesia in patients who desire it, we prefer local anesthesia with mild sedation. This allows the patient to communicate throughout the procedure so that immediate assessment of any neurologic change may be made. There are disadvantages to local anesthesia, however, and these include a higher likelihood of patient movement during the procedure with the inability to have complete immobilization during key elements of the procedure. This becomes most critical in situations in which "road mapping" is being used to guide the balloon angioplasty or stent deployment. Under most circumstances, however, patient cooperation is not a significant factor with modern anesthesia techniques.

ACCESS AND EQUIPMENT

Advances in equipment technology have resulted in the design and production of a variety of devices that allow successful percutaneous intervention. Balloons, guidewires, and stents may all play an important role in a procedure. The types and sizes of devices used during the intervention are dependent on the vessel to be treated and the access approach. At the Arizona Heart Institute, we have treated brachiocephalic lesions via the brachial, femoral, and retrograde carotid access routes. A brief description of each access method and the necessary equipment follows.

Brachial Access

Brachial access generally uses a 7F sheath introduced percutaneously. The lesion is crossed with an 80-cm, 0.035-inch, angled hydrophilic guidewire (Glidewire, MediTech/Boston Scientific, Watertown, Mass). When an occlusion exists, a 4F or 5F angiographic straight catheter (MediTech/Boston Scientific) is advanced over the guidewire to allow safe and easy access through the lesion. The advent of hydrophilic-coated guidewires like the Glidewire has greatly increased the ease and safety of lesion traversal, and high-resolution fluoroscopic equipment ensures better positioning of all wires. Steerable guidewires add another measure of control (and cost), but in our experience, the nitinol alloy core of the Glidewire resists bending and kinking, which makes it functionally identical to the steerable wires in all but the most circuitous vessels.

The angioplasty balloon (usual sizes range from 4 to 9 mm) is used for dilatation of the lesion. Balloon technology has shown remarkable headway in recent years as manufacturers strive to lower the profile of their products, increase their performance capabilities with new balloon materials, and overcome some inherently traumatic aspects of the traditional overflagged balloon design. The decision as to which balloons to stock is largely based on preference and periodic evaluation of new designs. For peripheral interventions, catheter lengths from 65 to 150 cm are commonly inventoried for a variety of balloon dimensions.

When we stent a lesion, we generally predilate by using a balloon that is one size smaller than the balloon the stent is mounted on. Selection of the stent size is based on the adjacent normal vessel and the length of the lesion. We frequently use Palmaz stents

(Cordis, a Johnson and Johnson Co., Miami, FL) or Wallstents (Schneider USA, Inc., Minneapolis). The Palmaz stent is available in varying lengths from 10 to 39 mm with expansion ranges of 4 to 18 mm. Its longitudinal rigidity and large diameter make it ideally suited for straight vessels. The Wallstent, however, is a cylindric device that is flexible, compliant, and self-expanding, which makes it an excellent choice for delivery through curved arteries and in vessels subject to flexion from adjacent joints or structures. The Wallstent comes in a variety of lengths ranging from 50 to 150 mm and in diameters from 5 to 10 mm.

Several advantages are apparent with the retrograde brachial approach. The distance between the access site and the lesion is short, and problems with tortuosity of the arch vessels are eliminated. Additionally, the brachial artery sheath can be attached to a pressure transducer for monitoring the pressure gradient so that its elimination may be documented after successful stent deployment. Failure to eliminate the pressure gradient is usually an indication for the use of a larger balloon to better expand the stent. Another possibility is that the lesion, particularly the portion at the aortic arch position, has not been completely covered with the stent.

The value of the Palmaz stent is illustrated in Figure 1, where a short occlusion of the left subclavian artery is treated with angioplasty and stent development. In situations in which the artery is occluded, angioplasty can still be performed in most cases. The problem of passing the retrograde wire to access the lesion can be obviated by selection of a 4F or 5F guiding catheter positioned coaxially in the lesion. The catheter permits the wire to be pushed forward through the more central portion of the obstructive atheromatous core and avoids subadventitial dissection.

In more complex and longer lesions, a flexible stent may be preferred. In some circumstances in which the lesion is exceedingly long, two Wallstents may be required to effect a satisfactory result. The flexible stent is preferable for situations in which excessive movement of the arm and shoulder is anticipated.

FIGURE 1.

A, retrograde angiogram of the left subclavian artery showing occlusion at the origin of the vertebral artery. The lesion is treated by catheter-directed wire passage into the aortic arch, followed by balloon angioplasty. **B,** Palmaz stent deployment ensures patency of the angioplastied vessel as confirmed by angiography.

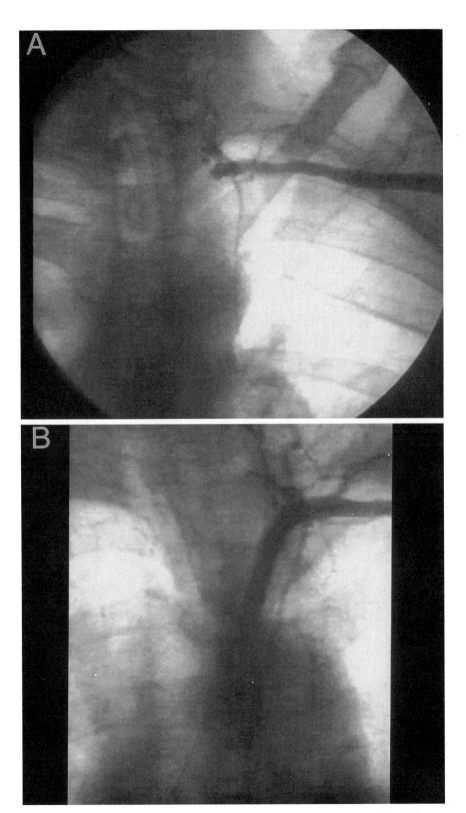

Femoral Access

Interventionists are generally most familiar with femoral access, and it has the advantage of entry into all of the arch vessel origins, thus permitting simultaneous treatment of more than one lesion. We place a 7F sheath in the femoral artery and access the brachiocephalic vessels with a JB-2 catheter (Cook, Inc., Bloomington, Ind); an angled guidewire is used to place the catheter in the origin of the appropriate vessel. Once the catheter is passed into the selected artery, road mapping is accomplished to enhance manipulation of the wire for access to the target lesions. The guidewire may be replaced with an exchange-length wire such as the extrastiff 0.038-inch Amplatz (Cook, Inc.) to provide better trackability for placement and advancement of a 9F guiding catheter (Cordis). Contrast is injected to allow determination of the dimensions of the artery and the nature and length of the lesion. In some cases, a guiding catheter may be omitted and the entire procedure performed through a 7F groin sheath. This determination is primarily based on the angle of the vessel originating from the aortic arch.

A balloon is selected for dilation, usually a size smaller than the anticipated final lumen size. In almost every case, balloon angioplasty is followed by stent deployment. The stent overcomes recoil, ensures that the plaque is compressed into the wall, and reduces restenosis. The balloon is inflated and a small bolus of contrast injected to assess the angioplasty result. In cases in which the lesion is to be stented, the balloon with stent is passed to the lesion. A second contrast injection is administered to confirm proper location unless road mapping is being used and the patient has not moved. The stent is deployed with a 5-second balloon inflation.

Retrograde Carotid Approach

Under certain circumstances, a retrograde carotid approach to an aortic arch lesion in the left common carotid, right common carotid, or brachiocephalic trunk may be preferred. The angle of origin of the aortic arch branches and the configuration of the aortic arch itself may preclude successful access from the retrograde femoral approach. We have used two retrograde common carotid techniques, one percutaneous and the other an open procedure.

In the percutaneous approach (Fig 2), needle entry and sheath insertion are performed approximately 2 cm below the bifurcation of the carotid artery. The wire is passed retrograde into the aortic arch, pressure gradients are confirmed, and the balloon-stenting procedure is accomplished. Heparinization is reversed, and the sheath is removed, immediately followed by manual compression of the puncture site for 15 minutes.

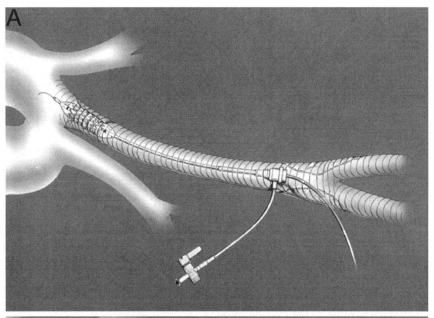

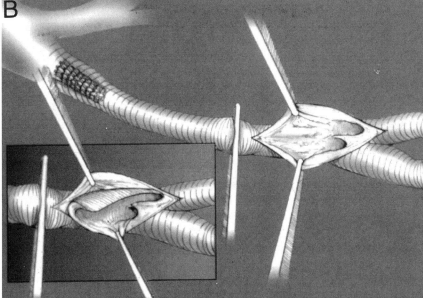

FIGURE 2.

Drawing showing the technique of percutaneous **(A)** and combined proximal common carotid stent deployment after surgical exposure of the cervical carotid artery **(B)**; this is followed by classic endarterectomy.

The open, or surgical, approach has been used most commonly for combined lesions at the aortic arch or in the midportion of the carotid artery and at the carotid bifurcation. Under these circumstances, a classic exposure of the carotid bifurcation is performed. The retrograde sheath is then inserted as though it were a percutaneous approach, and proximal stenting is accomplished. Clamps are applied, the sheath is removed, and an endarterectomy with or without patch graft angioplasty is performed. This combined procedure has been extremely useful and obviates the need for two separate procedures.

THE USE OF INTRAVASCULAR ULTRASOUND

Intravascular US (IVUS) is a useful tool in both the performance and assessment of these interventional procedures. At times, the exact location of a lesion at the aortic arch can be extremely difficult to determine by angiography. An IVUS examination can pinpoint the precise origin of the atherosclerotic plaque, and that reference point can then be used for proper deployment of the stent. In most cases, it is desirable to have a millimeter or so of stent extending into the aorta. Oftentimes, lesions arising at the arch contain plaque within the arch itself.

Intravascular US provides high-resolution, real-time images that delineate irregularities and ensure proper apposition of the stent against the arterial wall. Reassembled three-dimensional reconstructions are now available in a real-time mode. Images are presented either as longitudinal or volume views. The former are immediately available in the operating room and provide the physician an opportunity to make rapid clinical decisions after catheter pull-through. The use of specialized computer software allows the cylinder to be hemisected along its length for inspection of the luminal aspect of the artery (Fig 3).

At the Arizona Heart Institute, we have frequently used IVUS for preliminary assessment of the subclavian and innominate arteries before stenting. Disease is most commonly found at the origins and is well suited to treatment with angioplasty and stenting. When disease is present in the second part of the subclavian artery, angioplasty and stenting may compromise a patent vertebral artery. The use of IVUS here can define the proximity of disease to the vertebral artery origin. After stent deployment, IVUS is again useful because it is the only assessment modality that measures the arterial lumen and confirms proper apposition of the stent against the arterial wall. In situations in which the IVUS study indicates that the stent is not completely deployed (Fig 4), a larger balloon

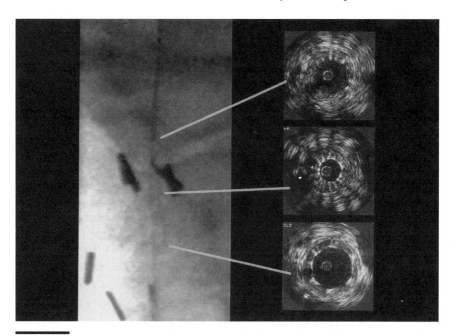

FIGURE 3.

Intravascular US study after deployment of a Palmaz stent in the proximal portion of the common carotid artery. The cephalad and caudal ends of the stent are perfectly apposed to the arterial wall. The midportion of the stent is incompletely expanded.

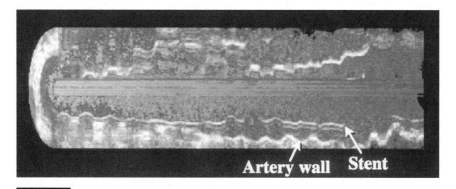

FIGURE 4.

Longitudinal intravascular US image of an incompletely deployed stent in the carotid artery. It is clear that the stent is not perfectly apposed to the artery wall.

should be selected and the stent more fully expanded—even in cases in which the angiogram appears entirely satisfactory.

THE USE OF ANTICOAGULANTS

A variety of opinions have been expressed regarding the preoperative and postprocedural use of antiplatelet drugs. We have not routinely used anything other than aspirin (325 mg) taken daily, and most of our patients do seem to comply with this regimen. During the procedure, however, the activated clotting time (ACT) is maintained above 200 seconds through the administration of heparin sodium. Between 2,000 and 5,000 units is usually given after the initial sheaths have been placed. If the procedure is a long one, repeat doses may be given. At the conclusion of the procedure, heparinization is reversed with protamine sulfate only if the sheaths are to be removed immediately. Otherwise, the patient is transferred to the recovery area, and the sheaths are removed when the ACT returns to the normal range.

COMPLICATIONS

Fortunately, the incidence of complications with these procedures is extremely low. The most feared complication, embolization with neurologic consequences, is seldom seen—probably because these lesions are not usually associated with loose debris. They are, in general, concentric and frequently quite calcific, yet they respond well to ballooning and stenting. The routine use of stents may also play a role in reducing embolic events and certainly decreases the adverse consequences of arterial dissection secondary to balloon dissection. Stents are also effective in overcoming arterial spasm, but again, in these larger vessels the incidence of spasm is extremely low. Recoil of the lesion is a more common finding and is easily resolved with deployment of a stent.

As with all angioplasty, the most frequently observed complications relate to arterial access. With the retrograde brachial approach, arterial spasm and even occlusion can occur after sheath removal. This is more frequently observed in female patients with small arteries. In some cases, we will approach the brachial artery with an open cutdown to avoid any complications after sheath removal. The usual occurrence of groin hematoma, pseudoaneurysm, and arteriovenous fistula (the latter two being infrequently observed) can be prevented by careful sheath removal and attention to the patient's coagulation status. Proper training of personnel in the recovery area is vital because they are responsible for care of the patient during the postprocedural period.

CLINICAL EXPERIENCE

Management of vascular occlusive disease is evolving as new technologies become available and new techniques are pioneered. Angioplasty has proved to be a valuable method of increasing luminal diameter in occluded arteries and has been used extensively in the coronary and peripheral arteries. Its use in lesions above the arch is more recent and has allowed interventionists to avoid open surgical procedures and their attendant risks.

It is clear that angioplasty has intrinsic value in the treatment of occlusive disease. But like many good ideas, angioplasty has spawned another important technology—stenting. The use of balloon angioplasty, particularly in proximal arch vessel lesions, is often associated with significant vessel recoil, and the interventionist may encounter calcium and atherosclerotic material that limit attainment of a stationary result. Deployment of a stent maintains maximum luminal diameter; stents are indicated in cases in which angioplasty yields suboptimal results and are now used routinely in many centers.

ANGIOPLASTY AND STENTING IN BRACHIOCEPHALIC VESSELS

Recent experience with angioplasty and stenting in the proximal brachiocephalic vessels has been described by a number of investigators.[4–8] In some of these reviews, interventionists have reported early experience with the treatment of carotid lesions as well.

In a retrospective study spanning 5 years, the records of 112 patients treated for 151 lesions in the innominate, subclavian, carotid, and vertebral arteries were reviewed.[4] The majority of procedures used standard retrograde femoral artery access and balloon dilation of the lesion site. Patients treated near the end of the 5-year period had stents deployed for suboptimal PTA. Procedures were considered successful when symptoms resolved and an increase in flow of more than 50% was achieved. In this series, 141 (93%) of 151 lesions were successfully treated. Treatment with PTA yielded a 100% success rate in stenotic lesions in the common carotid ($n = 8$), subclavian ($n = 67$), and innominate ($n = 13$) arteries. Three cases of periprocedural complications were reported, and of these, 1 was considered major. In this case, a focal stroke resulted in right arm weakness in a patient who underwent left common carotid PTA and stenting. Reocclusion was reported in 5 patients—all in subclavian vessels. The author concluded that PTA of the brachiocephalic vessels achieved excellent immediate and long-term results in proximal stenoses but cautioned that treatment of subclavian occlusions with PTA was likely to be less successful. This latter observation may prove less significant as techniques using catheter-directed angioplasty become more prevalent.

A similar retrospective analysis described the use of Palmaz stents in the treatment of lesions in the innominate artery ($n = 8$), left common carotid artery ($n = 5$), right common carotid artery ($n = 1$), and left subclavian artery ($n = 12$).[5] A total of 22 symptomatic patients (mean age, 61.3 years) were treated with 26 stents. Local anesthesia was used in 12 cases and general anesthesia in 10. In this series, surgical exposure of either the cervical common carotid or brachial artery was performed to allow distal clamping before retrograde stent deployment. Successful acute results were achieved in 26 cases (92.3%), and no strokes or deaths occurred. During a follow-up period of 27 months, 22 (85%) patients were asymptomatic with patent vessels. The authors concluded that stenting in the brachiocephalic vessels was an acceptable alternative to surgical intervention. Our experience indicates that routine exposure of the cervical carotid artery with clamping at the time of angioplasty is unnecessary and only makes the procedure more complicated.

Several investigators have reported their experience with primary stenting in the subclavian and innominate arteries. The deployment of a stent without initial balloon dilatation of the lesion may allow the operator to trap plaque and debris underneath the stent and limit the risk of embolism, which may be particularly important in supra-aortic vessels. The major problem with this approach is the potential for stent movement on the balloon as it is passed through a high-grade stenotic lesion. Prestent ballooning reduces the chance of stent migration and should definitely be used in cases with high-grade narrowing.

In a study of primary Palmaz stent implantation, procedures were successfully performed in 27 consecutive patients with 31 obstructed subclavian arteries.[6] A total of 50 stents were successfully deployed via the brachial ($n = 7$), femoral ($n = 16$), or combined ($n = 8$) approach. The percent diameter stenosis improved from 85% $\pm$ 12% to 6% $\pm$ 7% ($P < 0.001$). Peak and mean translesion gradients decreased, respectively, from 56 $\pm$ 35 mm Hg to 3 $\pm$ 4 mm Hg ($P < 0.01$) and from 29 $\pm$ 18 mm Hg to 2 $\pm$ 2 mm Hg ($P < 0.01$). Complications were minor and procedural; 1 stent migration was treated uneventfully with deployment in the right external iliac artery, and 2 brachial arteries required repair. The investigators concluded that primary subclavian artery stent deployment was very successful in the immediate restoration of pulsatile flow.

A separate series of 33 patients with lesions of the subclavian ($n = 31$) and innominate arteries ($n = 2$) were treated by primary

Palmaz stent deployment, with technical success in 31 of the patients.[7] Thirty of the 32 stented arteries (97%) were patent during a follow-up period of up to 2 years. Complications in this series included asymptomatic vertebral artery occlusion ($n = 1$), entry site hematoma or pseudoaneurysm ($n = 4$), and distal embolization ($n = 1$). The investigators concluded that endovascular repair of symptomatic lesions in the subclavian and innominate arteries was a viable alternative to standard surgical repair.

At the Arizona Heart Institute, interventions in the subclavian and innominate vessels have frequently included stents.[8] We recently evaluated the results of stenting of subclavian artery occlusions in 17 patients who underwent stenting of total occlusions in the subclavian arteries; 14 of these lesions were located on the left side, and 15 patients had a subclavian steal syndrome. The indications for stenting were vertebrobasilar insufficiency (VBI) ($n = 7$), arm claudication ($n = 5$), VBI and upper limb ischemia ($n = 3$), protection of a left internal mammary artery coronary bypass ($n = 1$), and an isolated subclavian steal syndrome ($n = 1$).

A total of 23 stents were implanted in 17 patients; 2 stents migrated during deployment for a 94% procedural success rate. One case of axillary thrombosis complicated our series but was successfully treated with local thrombolysis and balloon angioplasty; no postprocedural neurologic complications or deaths occurred. Follow-up over a mean of 19.4 months (range, 4 to 56 months) revealed 1 asymptomatic restenosis in a patient with 3 stents at 5 months. Life-table analysis showed an 81% cumulative patency rate at 6 months.

Stenting of subclavian artery occlusion appears to be safe and feasible with good short- to long-term patency. We have used Palmaz stents or Wallstents and achieved high implantation success rates. Successful treatment of stenoses and recurrent lesions has been realized in the majority of cases, and follow-up ranging up to 56 months with duplex Doppler scans and/or arteriography has confirmed patency in these patients. In general, we have preferred to use a stent after ballooning. In the case of ulcerated lesions, however, primary deployment has been used to prevent embolic consequences.

CONCLUSIONS

Treatment strategies for vascular occlusive disease have changed dramatically during the past 40 years, and balloon angioplasty and stenting are now in frequent use in the treatment of vascular lesions of coronary and peripheral arteries. Advances in catheter

technology have improved device versatility significantly and reduced complications related to access. Low-profile catheters that
can be accommodated by introducer sheaths that are 6F or smaller
are an important advance. New guidewires that allow the interventionist to cross lesions and occlusions with ease are also a valuable addition to the interventionist's armamentarium. Hydrophilic
coatings facilitate catheter passage, and significant improvements
have been achieved in the biomaterials of these new instruments.
Stent manufacturers are developing new and improved versions of
their devices as well, and more than 20 different stents are currently in clinical trials. It seems clear that technology will continue
to improve our ability to treat occlusive and stenotic disease via
percutaneous access methods.

Equipment advances have also included exciting break-
throughs in imaging techniques. The advent of IVUS has changed
percutaneous intervention significantly by allowing us clearer
delineation of vessel morphology and a means of assessing
adequate stent deployment. It is perhaps only natural that the
development of superior equipment and our accumulation of
experience with angioplasty and stenting in the coronary arteries
and vessels of the extremities have led us to the use of percutaneous techniques for the treatment of lesions in the brachiocephalic vessels.

Clinical experience with angioplasty and stenting in the proximal brachiocephalic vessels has proven extremely successful. Access via both the brachial and femoral routes has been favorable,
and complication rates are less than with classic operative reconstruction of these vessels. The goal of all percutaneous intervention is improvement in symptoms through restoration of adequate
blood flow. As endovascular surgeons, we endeavor to improve the
quality of life and offer treatment alternatives that extend its duration. Advancements in endoluminal technologies are now allowing us to offer less invasive means of obtaining these results in the
proximal brachiocephalic arteries. We are hopeful that additional
improvements in device technology and technique will allow us
to further our success in this arterial territory.

REFERENCES

1. *Heart and Stroke Facts: 1995 Statistical Supplement.* American Heart
    Association, Dallas, Texas, 1995.
2. Mathias K: Ein neues Kathetersystem zur perkutanen transluminalen
    Angioplastie von Karotisstenosen. *Fortschr Med* 95:1007–1011, 1977.
3. Tievsky AL, Druy EM, Mardiat JG: Transluminal angioplasty in post-

surgical stenosis of the extracranial carotid artery. *Am J Neuroradiol* 4:800–802, 1983.

4. Motarjeme A: Percutaneous transluminal angioplasty of supra-aortic vessels. *J Endovasc Surg* 3:171–181, 1996.

5. Queral LA, Criado FJ: The treatment of focal aortic arch branch lesions with Palmaz stents. *J Vasc Surg* 23:368–375, 1996.

6. Kumar K, Dorros G, Bates MC, et al: Primary stent development in occlusive subclavian artery disease. *Cathet Cardiovasc Diagn* 34:281–285, 1995.

7. Sullivan TM, Bacharach M, Childs MB: PTA and primary stenting of the subclavian and innominate arteries. *Circulation* 92:383S, 1995.

8. Martinez, R, Rodriguez-Lopez J, Torruella L, et al: Stenting for occlusion of subclavian arteries: Technical aspects and follow-up results. *Tex Heart J* 24:23–27, 1997.

CHAPTER 3

Brachiocephalic Arterial Revascularization:A Surgical Perspective

John W. Hallett, Jr., M.D.

Professor of Surgery, Mayo Clinic, Rochester, Minnesota

T his chapter summarizes current surgical strategies for brachio-cephalic arterial reconstruction, which will be placed in the context of an increasing interest in percutaneous transluminal angioplasty as an alternative to operative intervention. This surgical perspective is based on institutional experience at the Mayo Clinic, as well as a review of several major surgical series from other academic centers. The primary focus will be on surgical concepts and not operative minutia.[1–4] However, a few important technical tips will be emphasized.[4] Greater detail on this topic can be gained from perusal of several other publications relating our own experience and from the literature.[5–15]

A VARIABLE PATHOLOGIC ANATOMY

All the brachiocephalic arteries originate from the dome of the aortic arch in the superior mediastinum. In 80% of humans, the sequence of aortic arch branches is consistent. The first and most anterior trunk is the innominate or brachiocephalic artery, followed by the left common carotid artery and finally the left subclavian artery.[1] However, anatomical variability affects at least 20% of humans, and listed in order of increasing frequency are (1) close association between the origins of the innominate and left common carotid artery, 16%; (2) origin of the left common carotid from the innominate trunk (common brachiocephalic trunk), 8%; (3) origin of the left vertebral artery from the aortic arch between the left common carotid and left subclavian arteries, 6%; and (4) aberrant origin of the right subclavian artery from the aortic arch distal to the left subclavian artery and passage behind the trachea and esophagus, 1% (Fig 1).[1] For many patients, extracranial brachiocephalic arterial occlusive disease does not result in any symptoms because cervical arterial collateral networks are abundant (Fig 2). In addition, the likelihood of symptoms is influenced by the adequacy of the circle of Willis. In his classic review of 414 brains, C. Miller Fisher emphasized that 40% to 50% of patients will have some inadequacy in the circle.[2] In fact, some discontinuity of the circle of Willis between the carotid and the vertebrobasilar systems is significantly more frequent (78%) in patients with vertebrobasilar symptoms.

MAGNITUDE OF THE PROBLEM

Arterial reconstruction of the proximal brachiocephalic arteries is relatively uncommon in most surgical practices. For example, the Joint Study of Cerebrovascular Disease found an incidence of 17% for occlusion or stenosis of the subclavian, vertebral, or innominate arteries.[3] Left subclavian stenosis or occlusion was the most common aortic arch branch lesion. Of course, the presence of a stenosis or occlusion does not mandate surgical intervention; consequently, brachiocephalic arterial reconstructions constitute only a small percentage of all extracranial arterial operations (2% to 5%). Although current surgical approaches to brachiocephalic reconstruction are relatively straightforward and safe, the infrequent occurrence of brachiocephalic disease leaves many vascular surgeons with limited experience in this area and a heightened concern when such lesions are discovered.

A POTPOURRI OF FINDINGS

Disease of the aortic arch branches and the vertebral arteries can cause a wide range of symptoms and signs. Because many of the cerebral symptoms are identical to those associated with more distal disease of the carotid bifurcation, a thorough history and physical examination are essential to the recognition of clinical markers of proximal brachiocephalic disease.

The clinical findings can be condensed into *four major groups:* arm ischemia, anterior cerebral ischemia, vertebrobasilar ischemia, and combined symptoms.[15]

Proximal subclavian artery disease is the primary cause of *arm ischemia,* and in our experience, claudication is the most frequent manifestation (65%).[15] Microemboli from ulcerated plaque affect 20%, and the remaining 15% of patients complain of ischemic rest pain in the hand. Although most of these lesions are atheroscle-

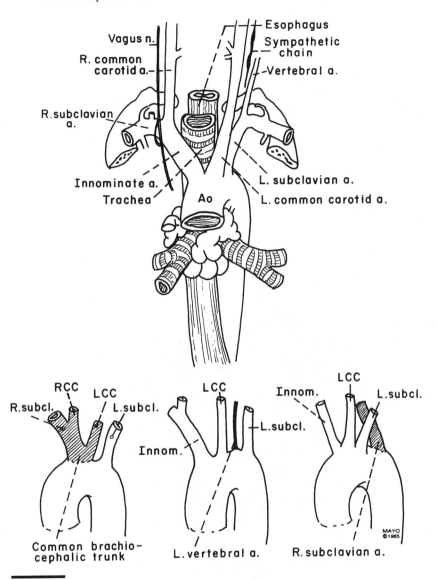

FIGURE 1.

Aortic arch branches and adjacent anatomy. Variance in the origin of the aortic arch branches affects 20% of normal adults. **Bottom,** a common brachiocephalic trunk **(left)** is the most common variant, followed by aberrant origins of the left vertebral **(middle)** and right subclavian arteries **(right).** *Abbreviations: n.,* nerve; *a.,* artery; *Ao,* aorta; *RCC,* right common carotid; *LCC,* left common carotid. (Courtesy of Mayo Foundation.)

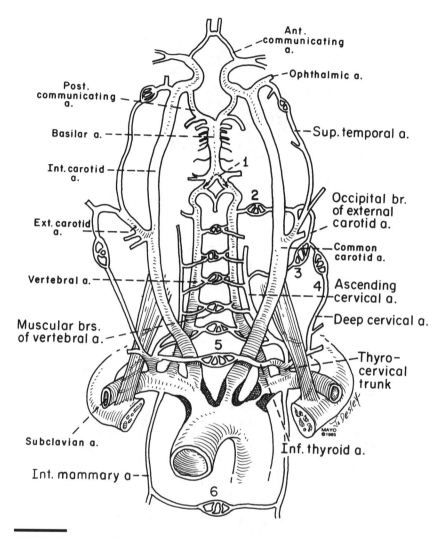

FIGURE 2.

Cervical arterial collateral networks are numerous: *1*, vertebrovertebral; *2*, external carotid (occipital branch)–vertebral (muscular branches); *3*, external carotid–thyroid cervical (ascending cervical); *4*, external carotid–costocervical (deep cervical); *5*, between the inferior thyroids; *6*, between the internal mammary arteries. (Courtesy of Mayo Foundation.)

rotic, two other common clinical problems requiring differentiation from subclavian arterial occlusive symptoms are thoracic outlet syndrome and Raynaud's syndrome.

Innominate and proximal left common carotid arterial disease can cause focal *anterior cerebral symptoms.* Nearly 85% of symptomatic patients will have high-grade stenosis or occlusion, whereas 15% have ulceration of a nonhemodynamically significant lesion. Symptoms from these lesions include transient hemiparesis, transient monocular blindness or unilateral persistent dim vision, or aphasia. However, severe innominate stenosis or occlusion may also be associated with a more generalized alteration in cerebral blood flow. These patients complain of episodic dizziness, vertigo, episodic binocular blurred vision, ataxia, confusion, decreased mentation, drop attacks, and syncope. Only 5% of patients with innominate disease complain of right arm exertional fatigue or have evidence of microemboli to the hand.

Vertebrobasilar symptoms generally occur in patients who have associated stenotic or occlusive lesions of the proximal vertebral arteries. In many of these patients, the circle of Willis is not intact with the anterior circulation.

Three primary physical findings should alert the clinician to the possibility of brachiocephalic occlusive disease.[4, 13–15] These signs include bruits over the upper part of the sternum, lower part of the neck, and the supraclavicular areas (85%); a blood pressure and pulse difference in the upper extremities (65%); and diminished carotid pulsation (40%). If both arm pressures are relatively low (80 to 110 mm Hg systolic pressure), it is helpful to compare the upper-extremity pressures with the Doppler-derived ankle pressures of the lower extremity, provided that pedal pulses are present.

In our Mayo Clinic series, 77% of the patients had neurologic symptoms when innominate disease was present.[4] Symptoms were referable to the anterior circulation in 50%, the posterior circulation in 40%, or both in 10%. In patients with symptoms attributable to the anterior circulation, amaurosis fugax was relatively common (60%) when compared with right hemispheric transient ischemic attacks (40%).[4]

DIAGNOSTIC EVALUATION

Although noninvasive tests may help in the diagnosis of brachiocephalic arterial occlusive disease, an arch aortogram with distal extracranial and intracranial views remains essential for surgical planning. Generally, we still obtain standard intra-arterial views. The role of MR angiography (MRA), especially with gadolinium enhancement, is still evolving.[16] In some patients, MRA provides adequate imaging. In others, MRA is simply not possible because of metallic devices in the chest region (e.g., cardiac pacemaker) or is intolerable because of claustrophobia in the MR unit.

Because noninvasive tests have been mentioned, their value deserves comment. Duplex US will frequently suggest proximal brachiocephalic occlusive disease by dampened carotid or subclavian waveforms, retrograde right carotid and vertebral flow in the presence of proximal innominate disease, or retrograde left vertebral flow in the presence of left subclavian occlusive lesions. If lesions of the innominate or left common carotid are hemodynamically significant, ocular pneumoplethysmography findings may be abnormal. We have not generally applied transcranial Doppler to such patients.

One must be cognizant that innominate artery occlusive lesions are often accompanied by other concomitant arch, carotid bifurcation, or vertebral artery lesions. In our Mayo Clinic series, 73% of the patients had multiple arch lesions and 12% had concomitant vertebral artery and carotid bifurcation lesions.[4] In Kieffer and colleagues' large series, 84% of their patients had an average of three associated lesions of the extracranial vessels, including 73% with carotid bifurcation lesions, 61% with subclavian artery lesions, 44% with common carotid lesions, and 43% with vertebral artery lesions.[5] Twelve percent of their patients had occlusion of the innominate artery, 70% had hemodynamically significant stenotic lesions (greater than 75%), and 18% had less stenotic lesions (50% to 74%) of the innominate artery. Only 16% of the patients had isolated lesions of the innominate artery. In the Texas Heart Institute series, 61% of the patients had multiple arch lesions.[6]

Arteriography can also help delineate the underlying etiology. Atherosclerosis remains the pathogenesis for over 90% of the patients with brachiocephalic arterial occlusive disease. In the remaining 10%, Takayasu's arteritis or prior head and neck irradiation will be causative factors. In some regions of the world, Takayasu's arteritis may be more prevalent.

DIRECT VS. EXTRATHORACIC SURGICAL APPROACHES

Both patient and anatomical factors will influence the choice of a direct or extrathoracic approach to brachiocephalic lesions.

Significant coronary heart disease is the most important medical co-morbidity that must be factored into the surgical approach.[5–8] If the patient needs concomitant median sternotomy and coronary artery bypass grafting, a direct approach to innominate or left common carotid disease is logical and convenient. On the other hand, some patients may have significant, uncorrectable cardiorespiratory medical co-morbidity where the risk of median sternotomy would be excessive. In such patients, an extrathoracic approach to innominate occlusion makes more sense, e.g., axillary-to-axillary bypass or subclavian-to-carotid bypass for proximal common carotid occlusions. Most operative mortalities in all large series have been associated with perioperative cardiac events in patients with significant heart disease.[4–12]

In patients with Takayasu's arteritis or other inflammatory arterial diseases, the current activity of the inflammation must be considered before proceeding with any operative intervention. Ongoing constitutional signs of inflammation and an elevated erythrocyte sedimentation rate should be controlled before operative intervention. Otherwise, grafts are likely to fail because of stenotic lesions that progress at anastomotic sites or in more distal segments of the involved arteries.

Anatomical factors also influence the operative approach. When the patient's health is excellent and the thorax is free of any previous surgical interventions, we favor direct approaches to all brachiocephalic lesions. For example, innominate and proximal left common carotid lesions are approached via a median sternotomy. Subclavian lesions are also approached directly via supraclavicular or cervical incisions for carotid-to-subclavian bypasses or subclavian-to-carotid transpositions. In contrast, some anatomical factors may mitigate against a direct surgical approach. For example, a patient who has had previous median sternotomies and an innominate occlusion may be a better candidate for an axillary-to-axillary bypass, a subclavian-to-subclavian bypass, or a carotid-to-carotid bypass.

The debate over whether brachiocephalic lesions should be approached surgically by direct or extrathoracic incisions is likely to continue. The availability of percutaneous transluminal balloon angioplasty with stents will only add to the dilemma.[17] Because direct brachiocephalic surgical reconstruction is currently safe in experienced hands and demonstrates excellent long-term durability, we continue to favor direct surgical approaches over all other methods.[4–8, 11, 12] Improved management of cardiovascular disease, advances in anesthesia, and better perioperative intensive care have all added to a less stressful experience for patients who undergo surgical reconstruction for brachiocephalic disease.

TECHNICAL TIPS

We have previously described the details of our surgical approach to various types of brachiocephalic reconstruction.[4, 13–15] Other surgical atlases are also excellent references. Nonetheless, a few critical technical tips deserve review.

INNOMINATE RECONSTRUCTION

After a full median sternotomy, the left brachiocephalic vein must be mobilized (Fig 3). If the vein seems to be in the way of adequate exposure, it can be safely ligated and divided without serious long-term sequelae.[5] Calcific plaque may make the dome of the aortic arch a treacherous place for a partial-occlusion clamp and anastomosis. Consequently, the pericardium should be opened to expose the softer anterior ascending aortic arch, which is most suitable for clamping and placement of the proximal anastomosis. In most cases, an 8- or 10-mm collagen-coated, polyester graft is used. Continuous electroencephalographic monitoring is used, and shunting is rarely necessary. In fact, the likelihood of cerebral ischemia can be minimized by maintaining relatively high mean blood pressures and occasionally by additional manipulation with anesthetic agents.

If *multiple* distal vessels are to be reconstructed, either a bifurcated graft or a single graft can be used. In some patients, a bulky bifurcated graft can be compressed by the superior mediastinal contents. If such compression appears problematic, a single graft limb can be anastomosed to the aortic arch with necessary side arms attached outside the confines of the thorax. However, the Texas Heart Institute has reported excellent results with bifurcated grafts.[6] They suggest using a long graft trunk with limb bifurcation placed high in the mediastinum.

We seldom use aorta-innominate endarterectomy anymore. It is only suitable for patients with focal, midinnominate lesions that do not extend down onto the aortic arch and do not extend into the subclavian or common carotid arteries. If one thinks that an endarterectomy may be suitable, it is mandatory that (1) the origin of the *left* common carotid artery be sufficiently far away from that of the innominate to allow clamping of the innominate artery without impingement on the left common carotid artery and (2) the arch

---

FIGURE 3.

Aorto-innominate grafting. **A,** a full median sternotomy with a curvilinear extension onto the base of the right side of the neck is the best incision for adequate exposure. **B,** the innominate vein can be mobilized or divided. Opening the pericardium over the ascending aortic arch generally exposes the relatively soft aorta for a graft anastomosis. **C,** the ascending aorta is partially occluded, and a 2-cm

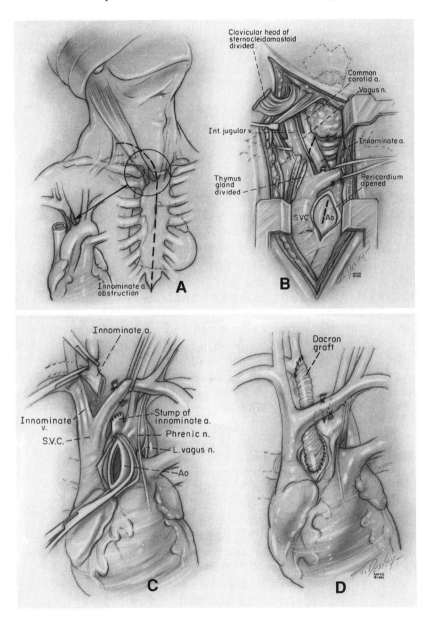

FIGURE 3. (cont.)

arteriotomy is made on the anterolateral surface. After construction of the aortic-canastomosis, the distal innominate artery is divided and the proximal stump oversewn. **D**, generally, an 8- or 10-cm polyester graft is used and placed beneath the innominate vein. A shunt is usually unnecessary.

of the aorta at the base of the innominate be free of extensive calcific plaque, thereby making both partial occlusion and endarterectomy safe.

We recommend systemic heparinization during innominate reconstruction. Also, the type of partial-occlusion clamp is extraordinarily important in gaining a secure purchase on the aortic arch. The Wylie J clamp has a relatively deep curve and was designed specifically for this type of operation.[10] The aortic arch must also be clamped so that cardiac outflow is not so restricted that myocardial ischemia occurs.

SUBCLAVIAN ARTERY RECONSTRUCTION

Carotid-subclavian bypass remains the most common operation for proximal subclavian occlusive disease, especially on the left side. Technical ease, relatively low morbidity and mortality, and good symptom relief are the main reasons for this current popularity. In exposing the left subclavian artery, one must be careful to avoid injury to the thoracic duct. This precaution is especially critical in patients in whom one chooses to perform a subclavian-to-carotid transposition. Generally, a 6- to 8-mm polyester graft conforms easily to the anatomy and has good long-term patency rates. If the proximal subclavian lesion has caused distal microthromboembolism to the hand, we ligate the subclavian beyond the ulcerated lesion but proximal to the vertebral artery. This maneuver prevents further embolization but allows continued retrograde subclavian flow into the left vertebral artery.

AXILLARY-TO-AXILLARY BYPASS

This solution to innominate artery occlusive disease is a relatively easy operation with negligible mortality and neurologic morbidity.[18] Although it is simple and safe, its durability is still in question. All clinical reports contain relatively small groups of patients with limited follow-up. The best estimate of patency is about 75% to 80% at 3 years, but one recent study reported 5-year patency rates in the 90% range.[19] Two potential disadvantages of this procedure must be considered: (1) its subcutaneous course over the sternum, which increases the risk of skin erosion and infection, and (2) its transsternal location, which makes a future median sternotomy for cardiac surgery a more difficult procedure. Despite these drawbacks, an axillary-to-axillary graft is a good choice for innominate occlusive disease in patients who are poor operative risks, perhaps for those who have had previous sternotomy, and for surgeons with limited experience with direct innominate reconstruction. We generally use either an 8-mm knitted polyester or polytetrafluoro-ethylene graft.

OUTCOMES

Outcomes must address two issues: safety and durability. Safety encompasses operative mortality and complications. Complications include both major neurologic deficits and local operative problems. Durability does not mean much unless results are known at 5 and 10 years.

Current operative mortality with transthoracic operations has improved in recent years and now ranges between 3% and 5%.[4, 14] Some authors have reported a high mortality rate, but most of these deaths have occurred in patients undergoing combined coronary and brachiocephalic reconstructions in the setting of increased medical co-morbidity.[7] Consequently, for good-risk patients with a reasonable life expectancy in the hands of experienced surgeons, transthoracic brachiocephalic reconstructions may offer a distinct advantage in long-term patency over extrathoracic procedures (Table 1). Mortality for extrathoracic procedures is lower and ranges between 0% to 4.8%.[15]

Perioperative transient or permanent neurologic deficits afflict 2% to 5% of patients undergoing both transthoracic and extrathoracic operations.[4–12, 18, 19] The stroke rate is not appreciably different from that for carotid endarterectomy alone. Stroke remains a common cause of major morbidity and death, especially in patients with associated distal arterial occlusion and in those with multiple lesions.

Local complications may involve cervical nerves or the thoracic duct.[15] Between 5% and 10% of cervical revascularizations are associated with postoperative dysfunction of the phrenic nerve, vagus nerve, brachial plexus, sympathetic chain, or thoracic duct. Patients must be informed of these menacing problems before surgery. With experience, these problems generally decline significantly.

Direct anatomical arterial reconstructions appear to have better durability than extra-anatomical grafts. For example, the Cleveland Clinic series noted a 3.4% late failure rate for direct transthoracic reconstructions as compared with a 9.1% late occlusion rate for extrathoracic repairs.[7] In another series from Crawford et al., the late functional results for all brachiocephalic reconstructions were encouraging: 83% of the patients were asymptomatic, 5.8% had transient neurologic symptoms, 3% had strokes but were alive,

TABLE 1.

Morbidity and Mortality in Published Series of Direct Surgical
Reconstructions of Innominate Artery Stenosis or Occlusion

Institution	No. of Patients	Perioperative Transient Ischemic Attack or Stroke, %	Mortality, %	Relief of Symptoms, %
Univ. of California, San Francisco, 1977	37	2.9	6	94
Cleveland Clinic, 1982	34	0	14.7	82
Baylor, 1983	43	5.5	4.7	94
Univ. of Michigan, 1985	17	5.9	0	100
Mass. Gen. Hospital, 1985	29	6.9	3.4	88
Ohio State Univ., 1988	26	7.6	7.6	96
Mayo Clinic, 1989	26	0	3.8	96
Texas Heart Institute, 1991	38	2.7	0	92
Pitiè-Salpétrière Univ. Hospital, 1995	148	5.4	5.4	92

and 8% died of or with a stroke.[8] Similar late results were reported
from the Cleveland Clinic. They also noted that about 25% of the
patients will eventually require another extracranial cerebrovascular operation, usually a carotid endarterectomy. In our own Mayo
Clinic series, 96% of the patients achieved relief of symptoms.[4]

The largest series of innominate artery reconstructions originates from Kieffer's work in France.[5] The probability of survival
was 77.5% and 51.9% at 5 and 10 years, respectively. In this series, 8.5% of the patients had late ischemic neurologic events.
However, there were no late right hemispheric strokes and only 1
late neurologic death in 148 patients. During a mean follow-up of
slightly longer than 6 years, 12% of the patients required reconstruction for disease progression. Only 1.5% of the patients had

occlusion of their innominate artery reconstruction, thus giving primary patency rates of 98.4% and 96.3% at 5 and 10 years, respectively. The secondary patency rates were 99.3% and 99.3% at 5 and 10 years. The probability of freedom from an ipsilateral neurologic event was 92.7% at 5 years and 84% at 10 years for a 1.4% annual occurrence rate (Fig. 4). The probability of freedom from an ipsilateral stroke was 98.6% at both 5 and 10 years. These long-term surgical results set high standards of performance for any new endovascular techniques.

FUTURE BRACHIOCEPHALIC RECONSTRUCTION

Surgical approaches to brachiocephalic arterial occlusive disease have become safer and more durable with time. For selected patients who have focal arterial lesions of the brachiocephalic trunks, percutaneous balloon angioplasty with or without stenting is another alternative, especially in patients with significant medical comorbidity. However, the results of such percutaneous therapy are likely to be temporary, especially when one examines results at 5 and 10 years. Currently, the best option for brachiocephalic arterial occlusive disease in good-risk patients remains surgical reconstruction.

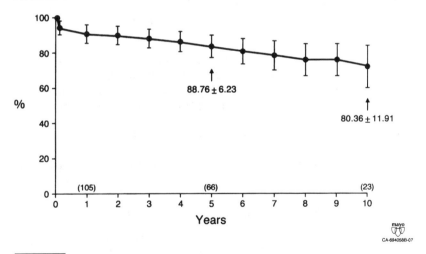

FIGURE 4

Survival free of neurologic symptoms after innominate artery reconstruction for arterial occlusive disease. (Modified from Kieffer E, Sabatler J, Koskas F, et al: Atherosclerotic innominate artery occlusive disease: Early and long term results of surgical reconstruction. *J Vasc Surg* 21:326–337, 1995.)

REFERENCES

1. Bosniak MA: An analysis of some anatomic-roentgenologic aspects of the brachiocephalic vessels. *AJR Am J Roentgenol* 91:1222–1231, 1969.
2. Fisher CM: The circle of Willis: Anatomical variations. *Vasc Dis* 2:99–105, 1965.
3. Fields WS, Lemak NA: Joint study of extracranial arterial occlusion: VII. Subclavian steal—a review of 168 cases. *JAMA* 222:1139–1143, 1972.
4. Cherry KJ, McCullough JL, Hallett JW, et al: Technical principles of direct innominate artery revascularization: A comparison of endarterectomy and bypass grafts. *J Vasc Surg* 9:718–723, 1989.
5. Kieffer E, Sabatler J, Koskas F, et al: Atherosclerotic innominate artery occlusive disease: early and long term results of surgical reconstruction. *J Vasc Surg* 21:326–337, 1995.
6. Ruel GJ, Jacobs HKHM, Gregoire JD, et al: Innominate artery occlusive disease: Surgical approach and long-term results. *J Vasc Surg* 14:405–412, 1991.
7. Vogt DP, Hertzner NR, O'Hara PJ, et al: Brachiocephalic arterial reconstruction. *Ann Surg* 196:541–552, 1982.
8. Crawford ES, Stowe CL, Powers RW Jr: Occlusion of innominate, common carotid and subclavian arteries: Long term results of surgical treatment. *Surgery* 95:781–791, 1983.
9. Brewster DC, Moncure AC, Darling RC, et al: Innominate artery lesions: Problems encountered and lessons learned. *J Vasc Surg* 2:99–112, 1985.
10. Wylie EJ, Effeney DJ: Surgery of the aortic arch branches and vertebral arteries. *Surg Clin North Am* 59:669–680, 1979.
11. Zelenock GB, Cronenwett JL, Graham LM, et al: Brachiocephalic arterial occlusions and stenoses: Manifestations and management of complex lesions. *Arch Surg* 120:370–376, 1985.
12. Evans WE, Williams TE, Hayes JP: Aortobrachiocephalic reconstruction. *Am J Surg* 156:100–102, 1988.
13. Whitley D, Cherry KJ Jr: Innominate artery reconstruction for occlusive disease. *Semin Vasc Surg* 9:84–92, 1996.
14. Loftus JP, Cherry KJ Jr: Surgical treatment of innominate artery atherosclerosis, in Ernst CB, Stanley JC (eds): *Current Therapy in Vascular Surgery.* St Louis, Mosby, 1995, pp 96–99.
15. Hallett JW, Bower TC, Cherry KJ Jr, et al: Brachiocephalic reconstruction, in Meyer FB (ed): *Sundt's Occlusive Cerebrovascular Disease.* Philadelphia, WB Saunders, 1994, pp 389–416.
16. Carpenter JP, Holland GA, Golden MA, et al: Magnetic resonance angiography of the aortic arch. *J Vasc Surg* 25:145–151, 1997.
17. Motarjeme A: Percutaneous transluminal angioplasty of supra-aortic vessels. *J Endovasc Surg* 3:171–181, 1996.

18. Lowell RC, Mills JL: Critical evaluation of axilloaxillary artery bypass for surgical management of symptomatic subclavian and innominate artery occlusive disease. *Cardiovasc Surg* 1:530–535, 1993.
19. Chang JB, Stein TA, Liu JP, et al: Long-term results with axillo-axillary bypass grafts for symptomatic subclavian artery insufficiency. *J Vasc Surg* 25:173-178, 1997.

PART III

Upper Extremity Ischemia

CHAPTER 4

Diagnosis and Treatment of Upper Extremity Ischemia*

W. Kent Williamson, M.D.
Resident, Department of Surgery, Division of Vascular Surgery, Oregon Health Sciences University, Portland, Oregon

Mark R. Nehler, M.D.
Fellow, Department of Surgery, Division of Vascular Surgery, Oregon Health Sciences University, Portland, Oregon

Lloyd M. Taylor, Jr., M.D.
Professor of Surgery, Department of Surgery, Division of Vascular Surgery, Oregon Health Sciences University, Portland, Oregon

John M. Porter, M.D.
Professor of Surgery, Department of Surgery, Division of Vascular Surgery, Oregon Health Sciences University, Portland, Oregon

V ascular surgeons grow accustomed to patients with symptomatic lower extremity ischemia caused by atherosclerosis; they have monotonously similar symptoms, patterns of occlusive disease, and appropriate treatment. In contrast, atherosclerosis is an unusual cause of symptomatic upper extremity ischemia. Raynaud's syndrome, a symptom complex defined as episodic digital color changes indicating ischemia occurring in response to environmental cold or emotional upset, develops in nearly all patients with upper extremity ischemia initially. These stereotypical symptoms result from a large variety of arterial conditions ranging from an exaggerated but benign vasospastic response, to cooling, to severe and extensive arterial obstructive disease. An understanding of how such diverse pathologic processes can produce

*Supported in part by Grant RR00334, General Clinical Research Centers Branch, Division of Research Resources, National Institutes of Health, Bethesda, Md.

Advances in Vascular Surgery®, vol. 5
©1997, Mosby–Year Book, Inc.

similar symptoms is essential for clinicians who treat patients with upper extremity ischemia. In this chapter we briefly describe the pathophysiology of Raynaud's syndrome and then describe the clinical and laboratory evaluation of patients that permits categorization into vasospastic or obstructive etiologies and large- vs. small-artery disease. We then demonstrate how subcategorizing patients into these groups facilitates diagnosis and treatment.

PATHOPHYSIOLOGY

All individuals experience spastic narrowing of the arteries of the hands and fingers in response to environmental cooling. The symptoms that constitute Raynaud's syndrome occur when this spasm is sufficient to result in complete arterial closure and cessation of detectable digital arterial flow with consequent digital *pallor.* When vasospasm ceases, the initial returning blood flow is rapidly desaturated and produces *cyanosis.* Then, as the dilated capillary bed is completely filled, the resulting hyperemia produces *rubor.* Many Raynaud's episodes do not include the classic tricolor sequence, either because they do not occur or because they are not perceived or reported by the patient.

In any individual, Raynaud's syndrome results from one of two possible pathophysiologic mechanisms: abnormal vasospasm or arterial obstruction. In *spastic Raynaud's syndrome,* the exaggerated spastic response to cold stimulus by normally patent arteries results in the cessation of flow. In *obstructive Raynaud's syndrome,* arteries in which digital pressure is already reduced by fixed arterial obstructive disease become completely obstructed by a normal vasospastic response to cold, and cessation of flow results. This means that the first task of the clinician is to determine whether patients with symptoms of upper extremity ischemia have vasospastic disease or obstructive arterial disease. It is clinically relevant to determine whether primarily large arteries (those proximal to the wrist), small arteries (those distal to the wrist), or, as occasionally happens, both (as when thrombus forms in a subclavian artery aneurysm and embolizes to obstruct digital arteries) are affected. The diagnostic steps that allow assignment of patients to these categories are described in the next section.

DIAGNOSTIC WORKUP

DIFFERENTIATING VASOSPASM FROM OBSTRUCTION

Table 1 classifies diseases and conditions that may produce Raynaud's syndrome into vasospastic or obstructive and specifies whether large or small arteries are affected. Knowledge of these di-

TABLE 1.
Associated Conditions and Causes of Upper Extremity Ischemia

Vasospastic conditions
  Small artery
    Idiopathic vasospastic Raynaud's syndrome
    β-Blockers
    Cytotoxic drugs
    Vibration injury
    Endocrinologic disorders
    Vinyl chloride exposure
  Large artery
    Ergotism
Obstructive arterial disorders
  Small artery
    Connective tissue disease
    Hypersensitivity angiitis
    Hypercoagulable disorders
    Malignancy
    Frostbite
    Embolization from a proximal large-artery source
    Buerger's disease—thromboangiitis obliterans
    Henoch-Schönlein purpura
    Mixed cryoglobulinemia
    Multiple myeloma
    Macroglobulinemia
    Thrombocytosis
    Polycythemia rubra vera
    Leukemia
  Large artery
    Thoracic outlet syndrome (bony abnormalities of the first or
     cervical rib or the clavicle)
    Atherosclerosis
    Fibromuscular disease
    Ulnar artery aneurysm

agnostic possibilities is a valuable guide to the clinical evaluation process and may lead to more efficient diagnosis.

Most patients with *vasospastic* Raynaud's syndrome are young women who have been symptomatic since their early teens, and both hands are affected equally. Ten percent of these patients complain of symptoms primarily in the feet or toes. In contrast, the obstructive Raynaud's syndrome gender ratio is 1:1, and most patients are older than 40 years of age. Digits are not affected symmetrically, and the lower extremities are infrequently involved. Patients with digital ischemic ulceration or gangrene always have obstructive arterial disease inasmuch as this problem does not occur as a result of abnormal vasospasm.[1]

Laboratory Testing

Objective differentiation of vasospastic from obstructive pathophysiology is best done with noninvasive vascular laboratory testing. The initial examination includes bilateral brachial, ulnar, and radial segmental blood pressure measurements, ten-finger photoplethysmography, Doppler analogue pulse recording, resting digital blood pressure measurements, and digital artery closure testing after cooling as described by Nielsen and Lassen.[2] These studies reliably differentiate obstructive (Fig 1) from vasospastic Raynaud's syndrome, localize the site of arterial blockage (large or small), and determine bilateral lesions in patients with unilateral symptoms. Digital photoplethysmography with digital blood pressure determination is as accurate as angiography in the detection of *significant* digital obstruction.[3]

Routine blood tests include serum chemistries, complete blood count, platelet count, antinuclear antibody, rheumatoid factor, erythrocyte sedimentation rate, and, on occasion, serum protein electrophoresis. Hypercoagulable screening consists of protein C, protein S, lupus anticoagulant, antithrombin III, lipoprotein A assay, antiphospholipid antibody, and factor V resistance to protein C. Hand radiographs are obtained in patients with small-artery pathology to evaluate for calcinosis or tuft resorption. Table 2 gives a complete list of laboratory tests to consider in any patient being evaluated for upper extremity ischemia.

DIFFERENTIATING LARGE- FROM SMALL-ARTERY OBSTRUCTION

In addition to obtaining the aforementioned upper extremity vascular laboratory testing, other tests may be performed to help differentiate large- from small-artery obstruction, which is important in directing later treatment. Upper extremity segmental pressure and finger photoplethysmography are initial tests that help distinguish the level of obstruction, and a chest radiograph should be obtained to identify the cervical ribs (Fig 2). The most common underlying pathology in patients with upper extremity ischemia from large-artery obstruction is atherosclerotic plaque in the subclavian artery, followed by subclavian artery aneurysms caused by bony

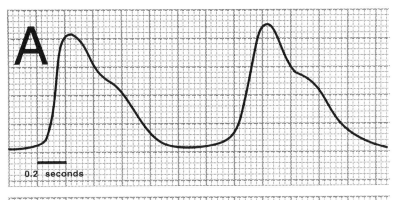

FIGURE 1.

Finger photoplethysmography demonstrating normal **(A)** and obstructive **(B)** waveforms. Note the blunted systolic peak in the obstructive waveform pattern. (Courtesy of Landry GJ, Edwards JM, McClafferty RB, et al: Long term outcome of Raynaud's syndrome in a prospectively analyzed cohort. *J Vasc Surg* 23:76–86, 1996.)

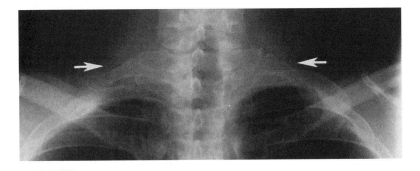

FIGURE 2.

Chest radiograph demonstrating prominent cervical ribs *(arrows)*. (Courtesy of Nehler MR, Taylor LM Jr, Moneta GL, et al: Upper extremity ischemia from subclavian artery aneurysm caused by bony abnormalities of the thoracic outlet. *Arch Surg,* 132(5):527–532, 1997.)

TABLE 2.

Diagnostic Evaluation of Upper Extremity Ischemia

	Routine	**In Selected Patients**
Laboratory	Complete blood count	Serum protein electrophoresis
	Urinalysis	Cold agglutinins
	Sedimentation rate	VDRL
	Automated	Hep-2 ANA
	multichemistry	Anti–native DNA antibody
	Rheumatoid factor	Extractable nuclear antigen
	Antinuclear antibody	Total hemolytic complement
		Complement (C3, C4)
		Immunoglobulin electrophoresis
		Cryoglobulins (cryocrit)
		Cryofibrinogen
		Direct Coombs' tests
		Hepatitis B antibody
		Hepatitis B antigen
Radiographic	Chest film	Barium swallow
	Hand films	Barium enema
	Magnification hand	IV pyelogram
	and upper extremity	
	angiography	
Vascular	Finger and toe digital	Digital photoplethysmography
laboratory	plethysmography	after heating and cooling
	Segmental upper and	Lower extremity pressure
	lower limb arterial	measurements
	pressures	
	Digital hypothermic	
	challenge test	
Other		Skin biopsy
		Muscle biopsy
		Arterial biopsy
		Oral mucosa biopsy
		Electromyelogram
		Nerve conduction
		ECG
		Schirmer's test

Abbreviation: ANA, antinuclear antibody.
(Courtesy of Edwards JM, Taylor LM Jr, Porter JM: Small artery disease of the upper extremity, in Machleder HI (ed): *Vascular Disorders of the Upper Extremity,* ed 2. Mount Kisco, NY, Futura Press, 1989, p 103.)

abnormalities of the thoracic outlet (complete cervical rib, abnormal first rib, or prior clavicular fracture), ulnar artery aneurysms at the wrist, and brachial artery aneurysms associated with a long-standing dialysis fistula.

Arteriography

Arteriography is reserved for patients with noninvasive tests indicating large-artery pathology and in occasional patients with *unilateral* small-artery pathology in whom a proximal embolic source is suspected. Angiographic evaluation should include the aortic arch to the fingertips, including hand magnification views. Hand warming, intra-arterial vasodilators, and magnification views are used as needed and may enhance the sensitivity and specificity of the angiogram[4] (Fig 3). The appearance of a subclavian artery aneurysm may range from dilation to luminal irregularity and occlusion and may be quite subtle (Figs 4 to 6). Bilateral studies are important for visualizing contralateral asymptomatic digital artery oc-

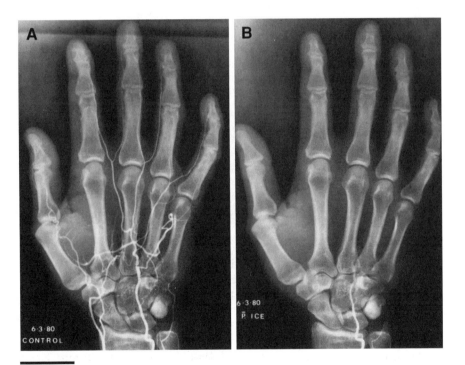

FIGURE 3.

Cryodynamic angiography demonstrating cold-induced vasospasm. Note the disappearance of the digital arteries after the administration of ice.

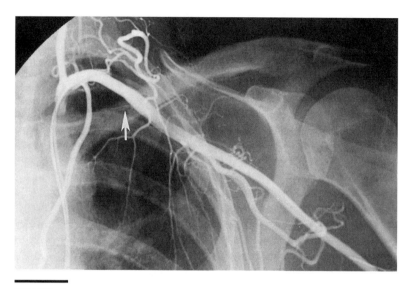

FIGURE 4.

Upper extremity angiogram in a 38-year-old woman with Raynaud's symptoms greater in the left than the right hand. Note the subtle enlargement of the left subclavian artery. Further angiography on this patient revealed a normal right subclavian artery and digital artery obstruction in both hands, indicative of an etiology other than the subclavian artery. Further testing suggested the diagnosis of rheumatoid arthritis. See also Figures 5 and 6.

clusions not detected on noninvasive evaluation (both common digital arteries must be occluded to diminish the plethysmographic digital waveform and digital blood pressure). This is particularly important for determining whether digital artery occlusions are from a proximal embolic source or a systemic process affecting small arteries in which only one hand is initially symptomatic.

PROGNOSIS AND TREATMENT

Once the diagnostic evaluation has established whether large or small arteries are affected and whether vasospasm or fixed obstructive disease exists, diagnostic testing can be concentrated into one of the areas listed in Table 1.

SMALL-ARTERY PATHOLOGY

Patients with a normal pulse and pressure at the elbow and wrist who have Raynaud's symptoms have small-artery pathology (confined to the hand). It is convenient to divide patients with small-artery pathology into four groups based on whether vasospasm or

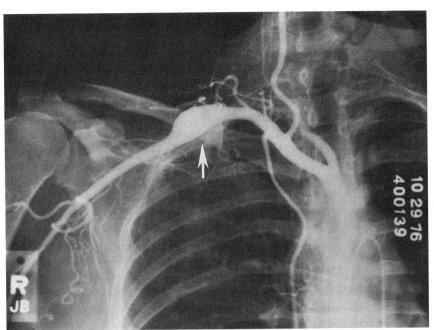

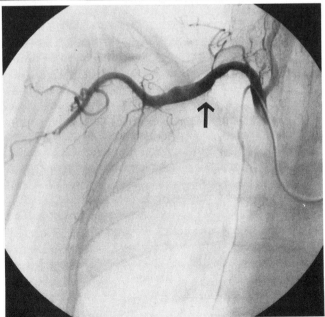

FIGURE 5.

Right upper extremity angiograms demonstrating the varied appearance of subclavian artery aneurysms. Note occlusion of the axillary artery from an embolus
in the **bottom** figure.

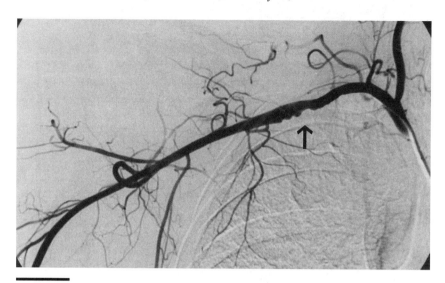

FIGURE 6.

Right upper extremity angiogram demonstrating a subclavian artery aneurysm with an irregular lumen, consistent with extensive thrombus formation.

obstruction exists and whether serologic screening for associated connective tissue disorders is positive or negative (Table 3). When a connective tissue disorder is suspected, rheumatologic consultation is obtained, with appropriate further specific testing performed to permit connective tissue disease diagnosis according to American Rheumatologic Association criteria.[5–9]

Small-Artery Disease—Vasospasm

Patients who have small-artery vasospasm with positive serologic screening have a high incidence of associated connective tissue disorders at diagnosis or follow-up, as demonstrated in Tables 3 and 4. Conversely, patients who have vasospasm with negative serologic results almost never have associated disease and rarely require treatment.[10]

Small-artery vasospastic disease is no more than a nuisance condition in the majority of patients, but for some, the symptoms may be severe enough to warrant medication. Treatment consists of cold avoidance, dressing warmly, and occasionally calcium channel blockers (nifedipine, 10 to 30 mg/day). Other medications such as reserpine, iloprost, angiotensin-converting enzyme inhibitors, and serotonin antagonists have been used with anecdotal success in some patients with severe symptomatology.

Small-Artery Disease—Obstructive

In sharp contrast to patients with pure vasospastic disease, patients with obstructive small-artery disease frequently have progression of symptoms to include the development of ischemic digital ulcers. Digital ulcers develop in half of all patients with obstructive disease of the hand and finger arteries, regardless of the serologic findings, with 10% to 20% eventually requiring digital amputation (see Table 3). Of those patients with serologic screening indicating connective tissue disorders, scleroderma has a particularly virulent course, with digital amputation frequently required. Patients with digital obstruction who are seronegative include those with Buerger's disease, hypersensitivity angiitis, vascular damage from vibratory tool use, hypercoagulable states, or digital artery emboli from a proximal source. Patients with these conditions also are at risk for digital ischemic ulcers (48%) and amputation (19%) (see Table 3).

Treatment of patients with obstructive small-artery disease is difficult both because of the chronicity of the underlying condition and because of the absence of any proven direct treatments that reverse the pathology. Vasodilators, including calcium channel blockers and prostaglandins, are frequently used; however, none have proven to be effective.

TABLE 3.

Prognosis and Associated Connective Tissue Disease in Patients With Small-Artery Pathology

Group*	CTD (DX)	CTD (FU)†	DU (FU)	DA (FU)
A	49%	16%	16%	1%
B	0%	2%	5%	2%
C	73%	30%	56%	12%
D	0%	9%	48%	19%

*Group A: serologic (+), vasospastic; group B: serologic (−), vasospastic; group C: serologic (+), obstructive; group D: serologic (−), obstructive.

†Percentage of all patients in these groups who did not have a connective tissue disease diagnosed at the initial examination in whom a connective tissue disease was diagnosed during follow-up.

Abbreviations: CTD, connective tissue disease; *DX,* at diagnosis; *FU,* during follow-up (mean, 3.2 years); *DU,* digital ulcer; *DA,* digital amputation.

(Courtesy of Landry GJ, Edwards JM, McClafferty RB, et al: Long term outcome of Raynaud's syndrome in a prospectively analyzed cohort. *J Vasc Surg* 23:76–86, 1996.)

TABLE 4.
Types of Connective Tissue Disease
in Patients With Small-Artery Pathology

CTD	n (%)*
Mixed CTD	33 (11.8)
Progressive systemic sclerosis	128 (45.9)
Rheumatoid arthritis	21 (7.5)
Sjögren's syndrome	24 (8.6)
Systemic lupus erythematosus	27 (9.7)
Undifferentiated CTD	35 (12.5)
Unknown CTD	11 (3.8)

*A total of 279 patients with small-artery upper extremity ischemia: 90 with vasospastic and 189 with obstructive pathology.
Abbreviation: CTD, connective tissue disease.
(Courtesy of Landry GJ, Edwards JM, McClafferty RB, et al: Long term outcome of Raynaud's syndrome in a prospectively analyzed cohort. *J Vasc Surg* 23:76–86, 1996.)

Surgical treatment consisting of digital periarterial sympathectomy and cervicodorsal sympathectomy have been used, but positive benefits have been uniformly short-lived, usually less than 6 months.[11] these procedures are not used in our practice.

Patients with digital ischemic ulcers invariably have severe pain that requires narcotics for even partial relief. Because of the distressing symptoms, patients and physicians alike may be tempted to proceed with digital amputation once ischemic ulcers occur. This practice should be avoided because fewer than half of the patients in whom digital ischemic ulcers develop ever require amputation (Tables 3 and 5). The natural history of digital ischemic ulceration in most patients is one of gradual resolution over weeks to months, followed by long periods of Raynaud's symptomatology only. Serial angiographic studies have shown that the development of collaterals rather than resolution of arterial obstruction appears to be responsible for the improvement.

Because most digital ulcers heal, treatment should be conservative, with amputation reserved for portions of digits that are frankly gangrenous. Conservative management includes careful cleansing, protective bandaging, and most important and most difficult, pain management. It is appropriate and necessary to prescribe adequate analgesia during periods of ischemic ulceration, and severe episodes may even require hospital admission and parenteral narcotics. In addition, many digital ischemic ulcers become infected, thus requiring antibiotic treatment. With these measures, most digital ulcers eventually heal. Besides these measures, the most important factor that influences healing is cigarette smoking. When ischemic ulcers occur in smokers who cannot stop, healing is rare. However, for those who successfully stop smoking, healing is the rule and digital amputations are vanishingly rare.

Ulcers that become gangrenous are treated by partial digital amputation, an outpatient procedure performed with local digital block anesthesia. Amputation is carried out through the midportion of the most distal unaffected phalanx.

LARGE-ARTERY PATHOLOGY

Most patients with large-artery pathology have abnormalities in upper extremity pulses and in segmental blood pressure at the elbow and wrist. Obstructive Raynaud's symptoms occur because of digital artery embolization either from a proximal source or from severe proximal arterial occlusion. In the following sections, the prognosis and treatment of vasospastic and obstructive large-artery disease are described.

Large-Artery Disease—Vasospastic

Vasospasm of large arteries is rare, and ergotism is the best described etiology. Ergotamines stimulate the contraction of vas-

---

TABLE 5.
Requirement for Digital or Phalangeal Amputation*

Classification	All Patients	Follow-up >10 yr
Spast, sero −	1.6%	6.3%
Spast, sero +	1.4%	0%
Obst, sero −	19.0%	25.0%
Obst, sero +	11.6%	20.0%

*Percentage of patients requiring digital amputation stratified according to vasospastic or obstructive pathology and serologic status.
(Courtesy of Landry GJ, Edwards JM, McClafferty RB, et al: Long term outcome of Raynaud's syndrome in a prospectively analyzed cohort. *J Vasc Surg* 23:76–86, 1996.)

cular smooth muscle and can produce damage to the vascular endothelium. Ergot-induced endothelial damage occasionally leads to thrombus formation, which may exacerbate large-artery obstruction. Large-artery vasospasm triggered by ergot appears as a tapered string on angiography, and rapid resolution of this tapered-string appearance after vasodilator administration helps confirm the diagnosis of ergotism.[12] The primary treatment is abstinence from ergotamines. In patients with severe symptoms, IV nitroprusside has resulted in rapid angiographic and clinical improvement.[12]

Large-Artery Disease—Obstructive

In contrast to small-artery disease, the conditions listed in Table 1 that cause large-artery obstruction are correctable by surgery. The excellent collateral blood supply in the upper extremity means that patients typically seek treatment only after disease is advanced and multiple occlusions exist. This is true both for proximal arterial obstructive disease such as that caused by atherosclerosis and rarely fibromuscular disease and for that caused by embolization from subclavian or ulnar artery aneurysms.

Diagnosis of the cause of large-artery obstruction is most readily made by arteriography, which should be performed in all patients with symptoms and noninvasive test results that point to a large-artery cause. Arteriography should also be performed in patients with noninvasive tests showing *unilateral* small-artery obstruction to detect proximal embolic sources that may not be producing detectable proximal obstruction.

For most patients with atherosclerotic occlusion of the subclavian artery, symptoms are minimal and surgical treatment is not required. For a few unusual patients whose occupational or avocational activities produce severe symptoms, subclavian-to-carotid transposition and carotid-to-subclavian bypass are satisfactory operations. Vertebrobasilar ischemic symptoms in patients with vertebral artery flow reversal are very rare but, when they occur, are an indication for surgery.

Some patients with subclavian artery *stenosis* collect thrombus at the site of the stenosis, which embolizes distally to occlude forearm and hand arteries and produce symptoms. Similar symptoms are produced when subclavian or ulnar artery aneurysms are the source of emboli.

In our experience, most patients with severe ischemic symptoms from distal emboli have extensive and multiple arterial occlusions, and it is tempting to consider thrombolytic therapy before arterial reconstruction. However, in our experience, this has rarely been of benefit. Exploration of arteries in which lysis has failed has shown chronic laminated fibrous thrombus with intraluminal synechiae. It seems apparent from these findings that most patients have had many episodes of embolization that remained asymptomatic until a final critical episode interrupted important collaterals and symptoms resulted. For these reasons, we prefer excision and interposition graft replacement of embolic sources combined with appropriate distal bypass grafting as required, regardless of the location of the embolic source.

Embolic occlusion of digital arteries from aneurysmal degeneration of the ulnar artery has been called "hypothenar hammer syndrome" because it typically occurs in patients whose occupations (mechanics, tire shop workers, carpenters) involve striking with the hand as though it were a hammer (Fig 7). Interestingly, 3 of the 15 ulnar artery aneurysms we have treated have been bilateral, including some patients who had no history of typical use of the asymptomatic contralateral hand.[13] This raises the question as

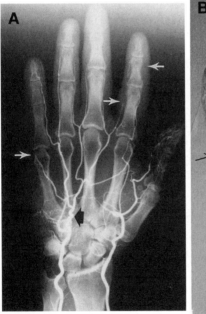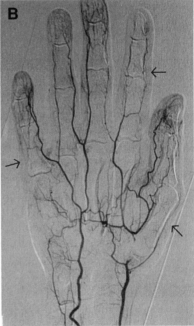

FIGURE 7.

Hand angiogram demonstrating a prominent ulnar artery aneurysm *(large arrow)* with multiple digital artery occlusions from emboli *(small arrows).*

to whether ulnar artery aneurysm is a congenital lesion that only becomes symptomatic in individuals who occupationally abuse their hands. Regardless of the nature of the arterial lesion of the distal radial and ulnar arteries (aneurysm or occlusive disease), autogenous vein bypass in a proximal-to-distal direction to the wrist has been a useful procedure. The site for distal anastomosis can be the distal extreme of the ulnar or radial arteries or either of the palmar arches, as indicated by arteriographic findings.

We have reported 17 arterial bypasses distal to the wrist in 15 patients with digital ischemia.[13] Ten had false or true aneurysms of the ulnar artery and 5 patients had end-stage renal disease with widespread forearm and hand arterial occlusions. Sixteen of the 17 grafts remained patent over a mean follow-up of 14 months. All patients with ulnar artery aneurysms had relief of rest pain. One patient with end-stage renal disease required digital amputation, and 1 patient required hand amputation, both of whom were initially seen with advanced digital gangrene. Interestingly, none of the patients with end-stage renal disease lived beyond 6 months, thus emphasizing that severe hand ischemia appears to be an end-stage manifestation of this disease.

Twelve patients with upper extremity ischemia as a result of embolism from a subclavian artery aneurysm have been treated at Oregon Health Science University in the past 16 years.[14] All patients had bony abnormalities of the thoracic outlet (eight cervical ribs, three abnormal first ribs, one clavicle fracture). All patients underwent bony resection, aneurysm excision, and interposition saphenous vein grafting performed by using combined simultaneous supraclavicular and infraclavicular incisions, and 8 patients underwent additional autogenous distal bypasses to the brachial or forearm arteries. During a mean follow-up of 18 months, all subclavian grafts remained patent. Two distal bypasses occluded, both in patients with preoperative arteriograms demonstrating no patent forearm arteries. Eleven of the 12 patients have had continuous symptomatic improvement, and only 1 patient has required digital amputation associated with distal bypass graft occlusion.

REFERENCES

1. Edwards JM, Taylor LM Jr, Porter JM: Small artery disease of the upper extremity, in Machleder HI (ed): *Vascular Disorders of the Upper Extremity,* ed 2. Mount Kisco, NY, Futura Press, 1989, p 103.
2. Nielsen SL, Lassen NA: Measurement of digital blood pressure after local cooling. *J Appl Physiol* 43:907–910, 1977.

3. Holmgren K, Baur GM, Porter JM: The role of digital photoplethys-mography in the evaluation of Raynaud's syndrome. *Bruit* 5:19, 1981.
4. Rosch J, Porter JM, Gralino B: Cryodynamic hand angiography in the diagnosis and management of Raynaud's syndrome. *Circulation* 55:807–810, 1977.
5. Tan EM, Cohen AS, Fries JF, et al: The 1982 revised criteria for the classification of systemic lupus erythematosus. *Arthritis Rheum* 25:271–277, 1982.
6. Mikerji B, Hardin JG: Undifferentiated, overlapping, and mixed con-nective tissue diseases. *Am J Med Sci* 305:114–119, 1993.
7. Fox RI, Saito I: Criteria for diagnosis of Sjögren's syndrome. *Rheum Dis Clin North Am* 20:391–407, 1994.
8. Rodnan GP, Jablonska S, Medsger TA Jr: Classification and nomencla-ture of progressive systemic sclerosis (scleroderma). *Clin Rheum Dis* 5:5–9, 1979.
9. Arnett FC, Edworthy SM, Bloch DA, et al: The American Rheumatism Association 1987 revised criteria for the classification of rheumatoid arthritis. *Arthritis Rheum* 31:315–324, 1988.
10. Landry GJ, Edwards JM, McLafferty RB, et al: Long-term outcome of Raynaud's syndrome in a prospectively analyzed patient cohort. *J Vasc Surg* 23:76–86, 1996.
11. Machleder HI, Wheeler E, Barber WF: Treatment of upper extremity ischemia by cervico-dorsal sympathectomy. *J Vasc Surg* 13:399–404, 1979.
12. Gomes A: Diagnostic and interventional angiography, in Machleder HI (ed): *Vascular Disorders of the Upper Extremity,* ed 2. Mount Kisco, NY, Futura Press, 1989, pp 59–99.
13. Nehler MR, Dalman RL, Harris EJ, et al: Upper extremity arterial by-pass distal to the wrist. *J Vasc Surg* 16:633–642, 1992.
14. Nehler MR, Taylor LM Jr, Moneta GL, et al: Upper extremity ischemia from subclavian artery aneurysm caused by bony abnormalities of the thoracic outlet. *Arch Surg,* 132(5):527–532, 1997.

PART IV

Access for
Hemodialysis

CHAPTER 5

Failing and Failed Hemodialysis Access Sites

Jeffrey L. Kaufman, M.D.
Division of Vascular Surgery, Baystate Medical Center, Springfield, Massachusetts

D ialysis techniques have undergone extraordinary change in the past 30 years. Initially reliant on external fistulas for hemodialysis access, dialysis patients have witnessed the advent of the autogenous fistula, the availability of a variety of prosthetic grafts when an autogenous vein is not available, the creation of new central venous catheters for temporary or long-term dialysis, the advent of peritoneal dialysis catheters, and the provision of new interventional radiology techniques for dialysis site salvage. With these have come vast increases in the quality and efficiency of dialyzers. These improvements have occurred under a system of expansive funding by Medicare. However, in the past decade it has become evident that increasing numbers of individuals are entering treatment for end-stage renal disease and survival while undergoing dialysis in the United States has not matched levels found in other countries.[1] These facts have forced reassessment of the quality and cost of dialysis care. Procedures for dialysis access account for approximately 25% of the hospital days for patients with end-stage renal disease, and most of these are for management of failing or failed access sites.[2] In an era of medical cost containment, surgeons are challenged to provide access sites that will function for a long time and, when failing, will be restored with the greatest efficiency.[3]

THE GOAL OF A PERFECT HEMODIALYSIS ACCESS SITE

Since the first clinical availability of dialysis, it has been evident that the efficiency of waste clearance is related to blood flow through the dialyzer. As dialysis equipment has improved, so have the flow volumes. Six- to 8-hour treatments at 200 to 250 mL/min, considered optimal 15 years ago, have evolved to treatments of 4 hours or less at 450 to 600 mL/min today. Therefore, the optimal dialysis access site delivers high flow volumes without mixing aspirated and returned blood (recirculation). The site must tolerate puncture three times per week without injury and must resist reactive scarring or stenosis from the high flow velocities at the return needle site. The site must have resistance to infection and to skin breakdown over the conduit. Optimally, placement of an access site would be inexpensive in resource cost and surgical time. It should be possible to place the site with minimal cardiopulmonary risk from anesthesia. The best site can be used immediately after placement to avoid temporary central vein catheterization. The ideal site lasts the whole of the patient's dialysis life without requirement for revision, treatment of obstruction, degeneration, or thrombosis.

Closest to the ideal site thus far is the Brescia-Cimino autogenous fistula from the radial artery to the cephalic vein.[4] I have observed such sites lasting more than 20 years with careful puncture by the dialysis staff and with flow volumes less than 400 mL/min. Autogenous alternatives include transposed basilic vein for the upper portion of the arm and saphenous loops in the thigh. Unfortunately, the majority of patients now entering hemodialysis are not candidates for autogenous access, largely because cannulation for previous medical treatments has led to irreversible scarring of either the vein or artery.[5] In addition, many of the very elderly or diabetic patients entering dialysis have significant calcification of the forearm arteries that does not allow dilatation to accommodate the increased flow volumes that an effective fistula must deliver. In western Massachusetts, autogenous fistulas now account for fewer than 10% of newly created access sites. In addition, as the percentage of autogenous access sites has decreased, dialysis nurses and technicians have become less experienced and more uncomfortable with them, which has led to a sort of dialysis "Gresham's law" in which some technicians have voiced their distaste with autogenous sites in favor of the easier-to-puncture prosthetic sites.

Prosthetic arteriovenous conduits have evolved in many ways over the past 20 years. The external Scribner shunt (and its femoral analogue the Thomas shunt) has been largely abandoned because its use is destructive to the native circulation, it has a high thrombosis and infection rate, and it is inconvenient. The demise of this shunt has coincided with the commercial availability of high-quality implantable artificial conduits, first the bovine heterograft, which still has advocates, and then the polytetrafluoroethylene (PTFE) graft. In the intervening years, a PTFE graft bonded to a percutaneous port system (the Hemasite) had been offered as a means for needleless access,[6] but it failed because of infection risk and cost. Multiple manufacturers of PTFE grafts now market grafts with interesting characteristics, such as external wraps, stretchability, thin walls, composite fibers, which may allow puncture for immediate use, and a tapered conformation, which may decrease the risk of vascular steal from the forearm; however, the benchmark for comparison at present is a standard-thickness PTFE graft. As a modern alternative to the bovine graft, there have been reports of human umbilical vein grafts used for hemodialysis.

STRATEGY OF LONG-TERM HEMODIALYSIS ACCESS AND ITS RELATIONSHIP TO FAILURE

Patients with new-onset renal failure will have ten possible regions for placement of an access construction: based on the radial artery; based on the brachial bifurcation in the proximal portion of the forearm; based on the brachial artery in the upper part of the arm; sited in the chest or neck based on the axillary, subclavian, or carotid arteries; and based on arteries of the lower extremities—each of these being potentially bilateral.[5] An access surgeon must create a strategy for a patient's lifetime of dialysis access, and no anatomical site should be abandoned without careful thought. One of the most important aspects of dialysis access surgery is creativity: how can a site be salvaged? Can the site be revised by inclusion of a segment of incorporated graft such that the patient can have immediate use of the site and avoid temporary central venous catheterization? The importance of this concept cannot be underestimated. In the early 1980s, prosthetic sites (PTFE) were commonly estimated to have a mean useful life approximating 2 years.[7] Recent experience in many centers, including those in western Massachusetts, has demonstrated a decrease in that graft survival. Because the goal of patient survival with maintenance hemodialysis is 10 to 20 years or more, there is a dangerous potential for a surgeon to exhaust all the major access regions unless care is taken to preserve sites for the future. It is fortunately rare for a patient to exhaust all access sites, but when that has occurred, the patient will become dependent on permanent central venous Silastic catheters, which will work in this role, albeit in a troublesome manner and for a limited period of time.

WHAT CONSTITUTES DIALYSIS ACCESS FAILURE?

Failure of dialysis access is not simply thrombosis of a site. It is failure of utility, i.e., delivering flow volumes that are inadequate to meet the patient's physiologic demands for dialysis clearance. The definition of adequate clearance remains a subject of intense debate by nephrologists, but it is clearly a function of the dialyzer as well as the flow characteristics of the access site. Clearance is reduced when recirculation is present. Recirculation can occur when flow volume in the conduit is restricted, either from arterial inflow disease or from outflow venous obstruction, such that the dialysis machine pumps and mixes returned (venous) blood retrogradely into the arterial or aspiration circuit. Sites should have a native flow volume sufficiently high that recirculation does not occur. Recirculation is therefore a function of the patient's arterial blood pressure, central venous pressure (which governs the resistance to venous outflow of an access site), the distance separating the aspiration and return needles, the luminal size of the dialysis conduit, and the flow volume of the dialysis machine. Utility of the site also means that it is used with conventional puncture by two needles, not limited by a threatened skin envelope; it is not indurated or inflamed by periconduit hematoma such that luminal placement is uncertain; the patient does not experience severe pain from its use; it is not causing ischemia in the extremity; and it is not threatening the patient's life through infection or hemorrhage. Sites with these characteristics are considered to be failing if they can be revised with urgent or elective surgery. Sites have failed when no resurrection is possible and a new conduit is necessary.

Should a site be repaired when malfunctioning commences, or should repair await unambiguous failure? From the standpoint of resource cost and ultimate outcome, no definitive studies have addressed this problem. No study has thus far demonstrated that dialysis graft thrombosis followed by thrombectomy and revision is associated with a significant decrement in long-term patency. The major impact of failure is its effect on dialysis continuity, and this is easily addressed with central venous catheters. It remains unclear from prospective studies whether vascular laboratory surveillance of grafts is cost-effective. The main rationale for the large expense of these studies is that early failure is certainly more conveniently approached with elective revision.[8] Nevertheless, the best indicators of early failure are a decrease in clearance or an increase in venous outflow pressure.[9] In general, graft thrombosis seems to be a sporadic event more often than not that is associated with factors that cannot be controlled by the nephrologist or surgeon, such as sudden hypotension or congestive heart failure, a technical mishap in the dialysis unit, or a careless action by the patient that places external pressure on the conduit. It is clear from these considerations that detection of a failing access site is an issue that needs to be addressed in carefully crafted prospective studies comparing current noninvasive technologies, clearance data, and outcome.

WHAT TO DO WHEN THE ACCESS SITE FAILS

GENERAL APPROACHES

Access site failure will often be determined by a dialysis technician, nurse, nephrologist, or the patient on the basis of a lost thrill or pulse. Occasionally this is an error in diagnosis, and a pencil Doppler probe will demonstrate that the site is patent with sluggish flow velocity. Sometimes, a pulse will be present but no flow. Accurate diagnosis is necessary because the immediate treatment may be different (balloon angioplasty) if the site is not fully clotted.

Optimally, the surgeon will have an opportunity to review the patient's access history when the diagnosis of failure is made. Here is the payoff for careful documentation of long-term plans for dialysis access and for detailed description not only of the site construction but also of any relevant anatomy or physiology that might affect future revisions of a site. When the site was placed, was the vein normal or scarred? How was previous revision handled, with simple balloon thrombectomy, with curettage, or with a patch angioplasty? In the last procedure, did the surgeon think that the site could be salvaged at the next sign of failure, or was it obvious that the next procedure should be a new graft in a new region? In the interval since the last procedure, has the site anatomy changed, perhaps with dilatation of new vein segments or progressive vascular disease? If one knows these answers, procedures will be more efficiently conducted. This process of communication must include the nephrologists so that they do not independently order interventional radiology procedures such as fistulograms, thrombolysis, percutaneous angioplasties, or even stent placements in sites for which a surgeon has already deemed these procedures to be unnecessary, futile, or inappropriate.

COAGULATION ISSUES

At the time of failure, the coagulation status of the patient should be discussed with the nephrologist. Has the patient been clotting dialysis coils? Does the patient require dialysis without heparin? Has there been a paradoxically low international normalized ratio or partial thromboplastin time? Has there been thrombocytosis? Was the clotting episode associated with inadvertent or planned cessation of an anticoagulant? Many dialysis patients are now observed to have a tendency toward hypercoagulability. The etiology of this is unclear, but it probably stems from chronic liver disease related to renal failure such that tests for common anticoagulant factors (protein C, protein S, antithrombin III) may show a diffuse, nonspecific decrease in levels, or there may be an acquired anticardiolipin antibody.[10] No series to date has related repeated site thrombosis to factor V Leiden (protein C resistance). Although there is a platelet aggregation defect in untreated uremia, it is unclear whether platelet dysfunction is related to this observed hypercoagulability. Even though some authors have expressed concern that erythropoietin promotes thrombosis,[11] presumably through an associated alteration in blood viscosity, no recent evidence has clearly defined higher hemoglobin levels with graft failure. In the majority of cases, the only observation relevant to hypercoagulability is that the site clots readily and frequently and this occurs despite multiple surgeons performing the access procedures. In effect, having several surgeons involved eliminates the possibility of repeated error in surgical technique as the cause of continued failure. These patients are usually managed with long-term warfarin, occasionally with subcutaneous heparin. Low–molecular weight heparin may play a role in the future. A brief course of IV heparin may be required after a thrombectomy while the warfarin dose is being regulated. In extreme cases of repeated thrombosis, the solution may be chronic peritoneal dialysis or conversion to dialysis with a long-term central venous catheter. For some patients, the best option will be a renal allograft, with the understanding that they may be at risk for early thrombosis of a vein or artery.

ANESTHESIA ISSUES

Careful documentation includes the choice of anesthesia technique. The goal of anesthesia is to facilitate an urgent procedure on a "short-stay" basis, following which it is often necessary to have the patient undergo dialysis in a geographically different location. Prolonged sedation is unwanted, yet pain must be controlled. General anesthesia for dialysis access is best reserved for the minority of patients who absolutely cannot stand regional or local procedures and for HIV-positive patients, where there may be less risk to operating room personnel by having fewer hollow-bore needles used during the procedure. Some surgeons prefer regional blocks to the arm, usually an axillary block technique. Other surgeons use local anesthesia with either 1% lidocaine or a mixture of lidocaine and bupivacaine, all without epinephrine. Brief, gentle sedation with propofol, fentanyl, or midazolam makes these techniques possible. It is especially important to note problems with dysphoric reactions and "release" phenomena under sedative-hypnotic drugs (where administration of the agent leads to paradoxical disinhibition and excessive movement rather than sedation). Finally, it is not unusual to perform dialysis access procedures on individuals with a history of opiate addiction or methadone treatment. These patients must be afforded pain relief in the early postoperative surgery setting without leading to conflicts over the administration of oral analgesics in the later postoperative period.

SURGICAL REVISION OF HEMODIALYSIS ACCESS SITES

The surgeon's responsibility beyond restoring access flow is to maintain dialysis continuity, which may necessitate placement of alternative dialysis access, such as through a central venous catheter, or the creation of access in a new site altogether. With local anesthesia or a regional block, the extent of surgery will be limited by the tolerance of the patient to remain still, which usually ranges from 2 to 3 hours. Therefore, a surgeon confronted by immediate and repeated intraoperative failure from thrombosis or low flow volume may need to restore dialysis access during a sequence of smaller procedures, with central venous catheterization used to bridge this period, rather than rely on one larger operation. To facilitate this, the surgeon must prepare and drape the extremity in a manner that allows immediate conversion of the procedure to creation of a new site in the same arm. This is easy for forearm sites, for which an upper arm field can be included; it is harder for upper arm sites, for which the high axilla or infraclavicular chest areas must be additionally draped.

Duraprep has become favored for skin preparation because of its lasting presence during surgery, resistance to washing off the skin with wound irrigation, and the fact that it does not act as a wetting agent (surfactant) on PTFE and lead to weeping of serous fluid under arterial pressure, as has been observed with povidone. Precise skin incisions are made with minimal use of cautery for hemostasis. Hemostatic clips are preferred because of their lessened tissue injury. Gentle self-retaining retractors similar to those used for tibial bypass surgery (Karmody retractor, V. Mueller/Baxter; Finsen or Mueller retractors, Aesculap; spring retractor, Codman) are preferred over sharp, tissue-tearing Weitlaner retractors.

Cautery must be avoided near nerves, especially for upper arm grafts where dissection is carried near the brachial plexus. Tunnels for new graft segments are prepared so that they are tight by using a bead slightly smaller than the graft (Impra tunneler). Hemostasis is precise, and hemostatic foam or mesh is not left in the wound if possible. All patients receive prophylactic antibiotics, either a cephalosporin or vancomycin, the latter being preferred because of its long duration of action in the presence of renal failure. Wounds are always irrigated with topical antibiotic solution. Skin closure is performed with subcutaneous absorbable material to close dead spaces, and subcuticular sutures with adhesive strips are used on the skin. New graft segments are first punctured approximately 1 week after placement, although with careful technique, immediate puncture at 24 hours has been done successfully.

The approach to thrombectomy is not a trivial issue. If possible, one should avoid graft incision in areas of repeated puncture, where dissection of the graft will expose puncture holes that may hemorrhage after restoration of flow and where suture of the weakened graft can prove difficult. In the past, a thrombectomy could often be reliably performed for loop access sites through a small transverse incision at the apex of the loop to facilitate passage of a balloon embolectomy catheter through both the arterial and venous sides of the construction. For uncertain reasons, in the past 10 years there has been a change in the pattern of thrombosis usually observed in prosthetic grafts—an accumulation of a heavy, leathery, white, laminated thrombus. This material is easily removed with a uterine curet or with new wire thrombectomy catheters. Associated with this phenomenon has been increased tenacity of clot at the anastomoses. To be certain that this material is completely removed, it has become increasingly necessary to open the graft adjacent to both the arterial and venous anastomoses. This necessitates two small incisions for broad upper arm loop or linear forearm constructions or reopening the whole antecubital incision for forearm loops. Although slightly more work, approaching the anastomotic areas under direct vision leads to decreasing numbers of grafts with recurrent failure caused by residual tenacious clot at the arterial anastomosis. It also facilitates revision of the venous anastomosis when severe intimal hyperplasia is observed.

The graft is approached by clearing the length between the arterial and venous side incisions and carefully flushing it with heparin-saline solution to remove all debris. Some surgeons check their work with angioscopy. Next, the arterial anastomosis is dis-obliterated. Patency of this segment is maintained either through systemic heparin administration or with regional retrograde heparin perfusion into the graft. Finally, the venous anastomosis is approached. It is best to avoid passing balloon catheters far into the venous system because this will cause an intimal injury that can lead to late stenosis. If there is no return of blood or if the balloon obviously traverses a stenosis, a critical narrowing from intimal hyperplasia must be assumed. The venous anastomosis is completely exposed, the outflow veins are clamped gently with low-pressure Yasargil clips or Silastic loops, and a longitudinal incision is made through the anastomosis. Minimal debridement of the intimal thickening is performed, just enough to be certain that flow will not lift a flap as it enters the vein. If the stenosis extends only 1 or 2 cm beyond the graft, the easiest revision is a PTFE patch angioplasty.[12, 13] Longer stenoses are often more easily approached by transecting the graft and interposing a new PTFE segment to a nondiseased outflow vein. In the upper portion of the arm, the brachial venous system adjacent to the brachial artery can be used to occasionally achieve new outflow by disconnecting and transposing the outflow to the second of the paired veins rather than interposing a new PTFE segment. Once the revision or thrombectomy is completed, the access site may require a few minutes to come to full flow. Palpation of the graft should not reveal a drop-off in pulsation, which may indicate a residual stenosis or clot. Intraoperative Doppler examination should reveal uniform flow without a high-pitched signal localized to a residual stenosis. Fistulography is rarely necessary in the operating room if the surgeon has a high index of suspicion that a thrombus is left in the graft and if such lesions are aggressively explored.

As noted earlier, hypercoagulability in the context of a failed graft is a significant problem. A few patients have been observed to have paradoxical persistent bleeding from suture lines after access revision, yet their grafts clot quickly, even in the operating room. The problem may be obviated to some extent if the surgeon uses PTFE suture because this may lead to less suture hole bleeding. Hemostasis at the anastomoses may require the use of topical surgical foam or cellulose mesh, both of which can be soaked in a topical thrombin solution. Systemic desmopressin acetate is also helpful. Because this phenomenon has occurred with systemic heparin doses less than 50 units/kg, achieving hemostasis is not simply a matter of giving protamine, which in any case may be counterproductive in the face of hypercoagulability. Careful hemostasis in this circumstance takes time and patience, even more so given the requirement of these patients to receive heparin drips until systemic anticoagulation with warfarin can be achieved.

CHOICE OF NEW HEMODIALYSIS SITES

When all the access sites in one extremity have failed and the surgeon turns to the opposite side, no definitive medical literature guides the surgeon in choosing the best initial prosthetic access site or conduit. Carefully constructed prospective and even retrospective studies with large numbers of patients have not been published in the past 10 years to define whether the linear radial-antecubital, forearm loop, or upper arm loop construction is best. Accordingly, each has its adherents based on solely subjective performance data. The initial selection probably does not matter as long as the surgeon does not squander sites because of poor planning or technique. Likewise, some studies have defined performance differences between grafts from different manufacturers, but in a prospective randomized study of linear forearm grafts at Baystate Medical Center, no substantial difference was found between Impra and Gore-Tex.[14]

In general, the "weak link" in construction of a new access site is the condition of the outflow veins. If one explores a site for a new graft and finds an apparently marginal vein, it is in the patient's best interest to place a graft there rather than totally abandon the site for reasons noted earlier. Although one can try to dilate the forearm veins with a proximal tourniquet as a preoperative test of venous sufficiency, the ultimate dilatation of these veins under continuous arteriovenous flow is impossible to predict. Small areas of early scarring from IV cannulation quickly become major venous stenoses after access placement. These problem areas can render a Brescia-Cimino fistula worthless for dialysis unless an interposition piece of vein or PTFE can restore high-volume flow or unless the arteriovenous anastomosis can be moved up the forearm. There is no consensus about the time interval during which an autogenous fistula should be rested for maximal venodilatation. Many surgeons have an impression that failure to dilate within 6 weeks indicates functional failure and the access plan deserves reevaluation. If dialysis must be instituted in that period, puncture of the site will only render matters worse. It is better to use a Silastic dialysis catheter until a decision can be made about the fate of the site. When the outflow of a PTFE graft fails to dilate, flow volumes will remain low. In addition, forcible stress from running high-efficiency dialysis too soon after the creation of such a site will invariably lead to thrombosis. Therefore it is important for dialysis staff to observe the outflow resistance in the form of venous pressure as a graft is used for the first time. If flows above 300 mL/min cause progressive increases in outflow backpressure, there is cause for concern that the veins are being damaged and clotting will occur.

Unusual grafts are considered for patients in whom the customary sites in the arms and groins have failed. Grafts from the midbrachial arteries to the axillary veins[15] have performed well, but grafts with jugular vein outflow have performed poorly at Baystate Medical Center. In extreme cases, grafts used in the form of "necklace" constructions between contralateral axillary arteries and veins or between the femoral and axillary vessels have been reported. These access sites will keep a patient alive for a short time, but they indicate impending loss of all dialysis access. They are themselves the indication for the dialysis team to initiate counseling of the patient on end-of-life issues. After all dialysis graft sites have been exhausted, dialysis can proceed for months with Silastic catheters, but these do not work forever. There will come a time when even these will fail and the patient will die.

USE OF CENTRAL VENOUS CATHETERS FOR HEMODIALYSIS

Central venous catheters deserve mention. The current urethane temporary catheters are less bioreactive than were the polyvinyl-chloride models initially marketed 15 years ago, and central venous thrombosis therefore seems less of a problem today. Nevertheless, venous scarring from catheters remains a potential issue, and it is best to avoid the subclavian veins if jugular veins are available. Silastic catheters can remain functional for months and are particularly helpful during the treatment of graft sepsis when all foreign material is removed from the extremities. When these catheters fail because of thrombosis, intraluminal urokinase will sometimes restore function. Otherwise, they can be easily replaced with a cutdown kit under local anesthesia in an office setting. When they fail to return blood yet allow infusion, the problem is generally a sleeve of thrombus surrounding the catheter. In the angiography suite it is possible to use a transfemoral catheter-guidewire loop setup to strip the catheter away from sleeve thrombus in order to restore aspiration. A major but fortunately rare complication with the use of dialysis catheters is septic central venous thrombosis, which requires removal of the foreign body, a prolonged course of antibiotics, and heparinization. There have been scattered reports of successful treatment of this problem with thrombectomy or vein excision in addition.

SPECIAL ISSUES IN HEMODIALYSIS ACCESS SITE FAILURE

The general causes of hemodialysis access failure are noted in Table 1.

TABLE 1.

Causes of Hemodialysis Access Site Failure

Conduit degeneration
 Aneurysms, false aneurysms, calcification, skin degeneration,
  bleeding, blowout
Infection
Anastomotic aneurysms
Perigraft seromas, lymphoceles, hematomas
Infiltration into the extremity adjacent to the graft
Iatrogenic failure
 Improper placement location, depth under skin
Steal
Improper use
 Incorrect needle placement, compression clamps for
  hemostasis
Edema
Carpal tunnel syndrome
Patient-related failure
 Hypercoagulability
 Phobias, pain from puncture
Flow abnormality
 Failure of venous segments to dilate, late stenosis of venous
  outflow
 Arterial flow insufficiency, proximal or distal
 Stenosis along the conduit with laminated white thrombus
 Recirculation
Loss of sites for further access construction
Cardiac dysfunction
 Hypotension, elevated central venous pressure
 High-output cardiac failure

ACCESS SITE PROBLEMS

Access site degeneration, a prominent cause of failure, includes loss of skin integrity, aneurysmal conduits, and mural calcification. The skin abnormality can be subtle—a small furuncle or excoriation over the conduit. These risk exposure of the conduit or failure of a puncture site to heal properly. The most ominous failure sign thereafter is bleeding, which usually heralds a more catastrophic failure as a result of either massive graft blowout or localized infection. The initial treatment of skin erosions is to rest that portion of the site; nurses must be advised to keep the lesion clean, dressed with a topical antiseptic agent, and free of adhesive tape. Further puncture of that site must be avoided. It is amazing how often a patient will describe repeated puncture into an area of obvious skin degeneration. If the degenerative conduit is still intact and the degeneration limited to a portion of the conduit, salvage is achieved by routing an interposition graft parallel to but away from the site in question. The old graft is left in place unless obviously infected or exposed. This technique has the advantage of retaining part of the original conduit for puncture to provide dialysis continuity. If the remaining segment is short, it is often still possible for single-needle dialysis to be performed for a few sessions to tide the patient over until the new segment can be safely punctured. After splicing the new conduit, the exposed graft or limited infected segment can be resected during the same operation, with care taken to seal down its subcutaneous tunnel. If drainage is necessary, closed-system, small-diameter tubing is used in the tunnel. In some cases, skin erosions exposing dialysis conduits have been closed with local rotation skin flaps, but these methods have not proven very successful in western Massachusetts. Patients in whom this complication develops always seem to have poor healing because of steroid use or malnutrition. In general, a primary graft repair offers greater security that the site will be salvaged.

GRAFT INFECTION

Major infection of a graft, in particular a recently placed conduit not incorporated into surrounding tissue, is troublesome and can threaten the patient's life from systemic sepsis and metastatic abscess formation. The solution is removal of the graft to the greatest extent possible.[12, 16] Invariably this involves sacrificial oversewing of the outflow vein. With only one failure in the past 5 years at Baystate Medical Center, a technique of subtotal graft excision has been used in which a small hood of the graft is left as a patch angioplasty on the arterial anastomosis. This technique is used when there is no abscess cavity or necrotic tissue in the vicinity of the artery and when the surgeon can find some adjacent soft tissue, preferably muscle, to pull over the residual PTFE hood. The only failure occurred in a patient with a bizarre *Mycobacterium* infection of a graft that ultimately required resection of the involved artery. Although some surgeons remove the length of an incorporated infected graft by completely incising the overlying skin, it is possible to avoid this mutilating procedure: a series of incisions are used to expose the graft, which can be removed through avulsion and sharp dissection to create a subcutaneous tunnel. The tunnel is then drained away from the arterial anastomosis with a closed suction apparatus, which is gradually removed starting on the second or third postoperative day.

In general, degenerative grafts without infection are left in situ when a new conduit is placed. Removal is invariably difficult and leaves an unsightly scar. Patients must be reassured that the old graft will lose its prominence and become a flattened, firm, linear mass. Late infection does not occur in such grafts. Leaving behind an aneurysmal PTFE segment containing a minimal amount of blood when placing a parallel conduit in a new tunnel has never led to infection in my experience. This same technique has also worked well when the old conduit is an aneurysmal bovine heterograft. In some instances, graft degeneration will take the form of graft wall false aneurysms. When these are small, 2 to 5 mm in size, they may be left alone, although the dialysis nurses must be cautioned to not puncture them. When these are larger, it is best to replace the conduit with a parallel interposition graft. The greatest difficulty with false aneurysms is the tendency to enter and disrupt them when performing a graft thrombectomy.

ANASTOMOTIC ANEURYSMS
Anastomotic aneurysms jeopardize an access site primarily because of skin erosion. The treatment is aneurysm resection with a technique that restores a smaller diameter and less wall tension through patch angioplasty or moves anastomoses away from the site of degeneration. This applies equally to arterial and venous anastomoses.

SEROMAS
Perigraft seromas noted soon after placement threaten the access site with infection because the graft, if punctured, will bleed into the subcutaneous tunnel. The etiology of seromas is uncertain. Low

serum oncotic pressure from hypoproteinemia with poor nutrition has been offered as a reason for failure of the micropores of PTFE to seal. An alternative and more likely explanation is surfactant material (povidone is an excellent example) causing the PTFE to lose its resistance to ultrafiltration of serum. If a seroma occurs and remains localized to an anastomosis, reclosure of the skin with clipping or coagulation of any visible lymphatics is a possible cure. Sometimes it is necessary to replace a short segment of graft found "weeping" fluid into the collection. Grafts totally surrounded by seroma fluid must be replaced within a new tunnel. Perigraft hematomas are not as dangerous because they can heal in time. Early hematomas will lead to fever, erythema, induration, or pain along the course of the graft. More than one graft has been removed for suspected sepsis and found instead to be encased in a sheath of sterile firm hematoma. Obviously, prevention of this complication is most important: it is best to use a tight graft tunnel formed well before any systemic anticoagulation is given. Late perigraft hematoma formation from aberrant puncture can lead to graft disincorporation, pain, induration, and hyperpigmentation. Continued puncture of such sites must be avoided. If necessary to achieve access site rest, a central venous catheter can be placed for 2 to 3 weeks. The patient is asked to elevate the site, apply a heating pad on low setting, and take anti-inflammatory drugs.

PUNCTURE SITE HEMATOMAS

Infiltration of venous return blood into the soft tissues of the extremity is among the greatest of dialysis graft catastrophes. This occurs with a through-and-through puncture of the dialysis graft. In seconds under active pumping, the patient can accumulate a profoundly painful massive collection of crystalloid fluid and blood. Although needle aspiration has been used in attempts to control the immediate compartment syndrome symptoms that accompany the most serious of these infiltrations, the best option is immediate surgical evacuation of the collection under local anesthesia and placement of closed suction drains in the residual cavity. A temporary central venous catheter should be placed contralateral to the affected side for dialysis continuity.

ERRORS IN SITE SELECTION

Dialysis site failure can result from error in surgical execution. A conduit that is placed excessively deep in the skin cannot be punctured cleanly, especially in obese patients. Sites created without sufficient length will prevent varied placement of puncture sites and lead to early graft failure from degeneration. Sites created excessively long may have a high impedance to flow and lead to increased thrombosis. Sites placed largely in intertrigenous areas, especially in the groin, may be difficult to puncture comfortably. All these problems are treated by interposing a new segment of graft in a manner that uses existing arterial and venous anastomoses yet corrects the placement site deficiency for the segment that must be punctured. In rare instances when there is no other site but the leg and obesity or lordosis obscures the puncture region, the graft can be replaced in the lower part of the thigh by basing it on the superficial femoral artery and using a tapered graft to prevent steal from the distal runoff in the calf.

ERRORS BY DIALYSIS PERSONNEL

Some aspects of dialysis access failure are related to dialysis center technique or policy. If the surgeon detects a pattern of repeated failure because of technique, the surgeon must personally intervene with an educational program. Dialysis center personnel undergo periodic turnover, which means that training programs and explanation of the surgeon's preferences will need to be repeated periodically. For example, every 1 to 2 years in some western Massachusetts dialysis centers, increased numbers of grafts have clotted for no apparent reason. Commonly, it has been found that dialysis technicians were again using clamp devices for puncture site hemostasis. Although the surgeons in this region have universally admonished the technicians to not use these devices, re-education has been necessary. Surgeons must learn to anticipate these problems, and this necessitates careful communication with the dialysis staff, especially when an access site differs from any institutional norms in terms of position, depth, orientation, composition, or ideal dialyzer flow volume.

PATIENT-RELATED PROBLEMS

There are a number of patient-related causes of relative or absolute dialysis access failure that may or may not be predictable before placement of the construction. These include the steal phenomenon, carpal tunnel syndrome, cardiac failure,[17] arm edema, puncture site pain from a cutaneous nerve, failure to achieve flow volume or dilatation of venous channels, and hypercoagulability. Several of these have the potential to cause limb deformity, dysfunction, or amputation. All demand that the dialysis staff notify the surgeon immediately after their onset.

A vexing but fortunately rare problem is a patient who finds the presence of an access site or temporary central venous catheter repulsive or who becomes indignant about the cutaneous scarring that is inevitable from repeated access puncture. All dialysis patients should have access to psychological counseling to help them cope with their disease, and phobias against dialysis or access must be addressed early and aggressively. Some patients also make unrealistic demands on the surgical staff about the conduct of dialysis access surgery. Obviously, any procedure is a matter of compromise between the patient's needs and the viewpoints of the surgeon and nephrologist, and physicians have an obligation to accommodate the patient with compassion, if possible. The problem occurs when patients make demands that either cannot be met, such as specifying the precise timing of emergency procedures for a failed access, or are unsafe in relation to their health while undergoing dialysis. Often, a crisis of personality, depression, or conflict with the medical personnel is best treated with a vigorous dialysis session through a temporary femoral catheter, which allows time for resolution.

ISCHEMIA AND VASCULAR STEAL

Vascular steal with the induction of significant distal ischemia has occurred with increasing frequency in the last 6 years. For unknown reasons, it was an uncommon event in the 1980s. Ischemic symptoms in the hand after initial placement of a graft or fistula are now common[18] and have caused many access surgeons to change their philosophy of access graft construction. The absence of a palpable radial artery is a common finding in patients with diabetes, who appear to be the population at greatest risk for steal from forearm access sites. When steal has occurred with a straight graft, narrowing the arterial inflow to the point where there is a Doppler flow alteration may help the hand.[19] Using the upper part of the arm as the initial site has not solved the problem if the conduit chosen is a straight 6- or 8-mm graft, but tapered 4- to 7-mm conduits may result in less steal. In a few cases, steal has been obviated by reversing the graft orientation such that the inflow comes off a larger proximal artery, presumably with a greater flow capacity.[20] In addition, the appearance of progressive steal over the first 6 to 12 months of maintenance dialysis has also become a prominent problem. Within that time period I have observed the loss of all radial, ulnar, and pedal pulses, and the reason for this aggressive occlusive disease is unknown. This population also has an ex-cess risk of major leg amputation because of nonreconstructible tibial and pedal vascular disease, and digital amputation in the hand is no longer rare. Fortunately, no patient has lost an arm because of this disease. Treatment has been to move the site quickly to an uninvolved extremity or to consider access in the groin, where steal has not been such a common problem. There have also been patients in occupations in which even the slightest symptoms of steal cannot be tolerated, such as musicians, and they have elected to have their primary access in the groin rather than risk their performance. Some patients with steal have required dialysis through a central venous catheter for life. Excessive dialysis-related mortality has been noted in this population. In the literature are described patients who have undergone arterial bypasses and ligations[21] or flow reversal procedures to counter steal, but these have not been very successful in western Massachusetts.

Global vascular insufficiency in the upper extremity from proximal lesions in the brachiocephalic, subclavian, or axillary arteries will cause repeated thrombosis and failure of distal grafts. It is not unusual to unmask stenoses in the proximal arteries that were not detectable by measuring brachial blood pressures. A hint of such a lesion is a palpable pulse in the brachial artery at the arterial inflow to the graft that disappears when flow commences. Treatment is inflow reconstruction, either balloon angioplasty of the inflow lesion or procedures such as carotid-subclavian bypass.

CARPAL TUNNEL SYNDROME

Carpal tunnel syndrome uncommonly occurs when access sites are based on the wrist.[22] The etiology is a stenosis causing a shift from direct radial inflow to inflow derived from collaterals in the hand and from the ulnar artery. Hypertrophy of these arteries leads to pressure on the median nerve at the wrist. Treatment of this rare problem is revision of the site to improve direct flow into the fistula. The other neuropathic phenomenon of interest is severe pain from repeated access puncture caused by irritation of a cutaneous nerve that unfortuitously resides over the conduit. In most of these rare cases, the conduit will require revision to a new site.

EDEMA

The incidence of arm edema from central venous stenosis has decreased in recent years. This is due to a vigilant policy that subclavian veins are to be avoided for temporary dialysis access catheters unless the ipsilateral arm is deemed useless for any further arteriovenous graft construction. Edema caused by a documented outflow central venous stenosis (primarily in the axillary-subclavian vein segments) can be treated by two possible approaches: stenting of the abnormal segment or bypass construction from the venous system at the level of the axilla to the jugular vein. If the access site drains into a large cephalic vein and has very high flow volume, the latter is a very attractive solution. The central veins are an "off-label" site for the application of stents, but the few reports of their use have indicated good results.

NONSURGICAL TREATMENT OF A FAILING DIALYSIS SITE

Fistulography and interventions to treat failing dialysis grafts are now the most common procedures performed by the angiography department at Baystate Medical Center and have supplanted historically common peripheral vascular indications. Unfortunately, many dialysis centers have established relationships with angiography departments that lead to unnecessary fistulograms and angioplasties for problems that are best treated surgically. A failing site should first receive expert assessment with a pencil Doppler probe instrument, which may clearly define a site of flow restriction. This can, if necessary, be confirmed by duplex US. When the flow problem is unclear after these examinations, fistulography is indicated. It remains controversial whether angioplasty[13, 23, 24] is a more cost-effective treatment than surgical reconstruction for stenotic lesions. Stenting intimal lesions at anastomoses does not appear to be worthwhile. Not only have stents failed to provide long patency, but any attempt at thrombectomy past a stent will be frustrated by repeated rupture of embolectomy catheter balloons. In addition, I have observed a peculiar inflammatory response to the outflow vein in the region of the stent. When confronted with a stented outflow site and a thrombosed access graft, it is my policy to move the venous outflow by interposition extension to a new vein segment or to abandon the access site altogether and construct one in a new region. Stents in central vein stenoses (axillary or subclavian) are a logical answer to the problem of rebound stenosis that occurs after balloon angioplasty in segments affected by intimal hyperplasia, and they may be very effective treatment.[25] At the time of fistulography, the angiographer must be prepared to measure pressures because central venous hypertension can easily cause failure, just as can an adjacent outflow stenosis.

Adequate numbers of reports now define the utility of catheter washout and thrombolysis techniques in restoring access graft patency after thrombosis.[24, 26] Recently created sites that clot because of a technical error by dialysis staff or because of patient maltreatment are among the best candidates for this technique. These are sites not likely to be stenosed by intimal hyperplasia at the outflow or to have large amounts of laminated white thrombus in the body of the graft. It is the treatment of older grafts with stenoses that remains controversial. Prospective studies need to define the utility of catheter techniques vs. surgery not only in terms of immediate restoration of patency but also in terms of cost-effective resource utilization. In light of managed care with reduced surgery fees, increased price competition among graft manufacturers, increased use of day stay or surgery center sites of service, and lessened surgical complication rates, thrombolysis and balloon angioplasty, especially when combined with stenting, may not be the best treatment of a clotted graft.

CONCLUSION

Dialysis access procedures have a huge impact in the scope of modern medicine: they are life sustaining to the ever-increasing population with end-stage renal disease. They involve a large hospital resource cost and demand much effort from surgeons, angiographers, and nephrologists. As with many other disciplines in surgery, dialysis access is most successful when performed by a group of surgeons who work together efficiently to establish standardized approaches to the problem with the greatest efficiency of effort. Dialysis access creation, failure, and resurrection demand careful attention and meticulous technique to ensure the highest quality of life possible for people with renal failure.

REFERENCES

1. Hellerstedt WL, Johnson WJ, Ascher N, et al: Survival rates of 2,728 patients with end-stage renal disease. *Mayo Clin Proc* 59:776–783, 1984.
2. Carlson DM, Duncan DA, Naessens JM, et al: Hospitalization in dialysis patients. *Mayo Clin Proc* 59:769–775, 1984.
3. Chapman JE, Sinicrope RA, Clark DM: Angio and peritoneal access for end-stage renal disease in the community hospital: A cost analysis. *Am Surg* 52:315–319, 1986.
4. Kherlakian GM, Roedersheimer LR, Arbaugh JJ, et al: Comparison of autogenous fistula versus expanded polytetrafluoroethylene graft fistula for angioaccess in hemodialysis. *Am J Surg* 152:238–243, 1986.
5. Kaufman JL: Revisional surgery for hemodialysis access. *Semin Dial* 9:41S–50S, 1996.
6. Jain KM, Patil KD, Grochowski EC, et al: The Hemasite-incorporated graft. *Am J Surg* 148:637–639, 1984.

7. Palder SV, Kirkman RL, Whittemore AD, et al: Vascular access for hemodialysis: Patency rates and results of revision. *Ann Surg* 202:235–239, 1985.

8. Sands J, Young S, Miranda C: Effect of Doppler flow screening studies and elective revisions on dialysis access failure. *ASAIO J* 38:524–527, 1992.

9. Besarab A, Sullivan KL, Ross RP, et al: Utility of intra-access pressure monitoring in detecting and correcting venous outlet stenoses prior to thrombosis. *Kidney Int* 47:1364–1373, 1995.

10. Chew SL, Lins RL, Daelemans R, et al: Are antiphospholipid antibodies clinically relevant in dialysis patients? *Nephrol Dial Transplant* 7:1194–1198, 1992.

11. Shinaberger JH, Miller JH, Gardner PW: Erythropoietin alert: Risks of high hematocrit hemodialysis. *Trans ASAIO* 34:179–184, 1988.

12. Corry RJ, Patel NP, West JC: Surgical management of complications of vascular access for hemodialysis. *Surg Gynecol Obstet* 151:49–54, 1980.

13. Brotman DN, Fandos L, Faust GR, et al: Hemodialysis graft salvage. *J Am Coll Surg* 178:431–434, 1994.

14. Kaufman JL, Garb JL, Berman JA, et al: A prospective comparison of two expanded polytetrafluoroethylene grafts for linear forearm hemodialysis access: Does the manufacturer matter? *J Am Coll Surg,* in press.

15. Bittner HB, Weaver JP: The brachioaxillary interposition graft as a successful tertiary vascular access procedure for hemodialysis. *Am J Surg* 167:615–617, 1994.

16. Gifford RRM: Management of tunnel infections of dialysis polytetrafluoroethylene grafts. *J Vasc Surg* 2:854–858, 1985.

17. Engelberts I, Tordoir JH, Boon ES, et al: High-output cardiac failure due to excessive shunting in a hemodialysis access fistula: An easily overlooked diagnosis. *Am J Nephrol* 15:323–326, 1995.

18. Tzamaloukas AH, Murata GH, Harford AM, et al: Hand gangrene in diabetic patients on chronic dialysis. *ASAIO Trans* 37:638–643, 1991.

19. Jain KM, Simoni EJ, Munn JS: A new technique to correct vascular steal secondary to hemodialysis grafts. *Surg Gynecol Obstet* 175:183–184, 1992.

20. Schlak JA, Lukens ML, Mayes JT: Salvage of thrombosed forearm polytetrafluoroethylene vascular access grafts by reversal of flow direction and venous bypass grafting. *Am J Surg* 161:485–487, 1991.

21. Schanzer H, Schwartz M, Harrington E, et al: Treatment of ischemia due to "steal" by arteriovenous fistula with distal artery ligation and revascularization. *J Vasc Surg* 7:770–773, 1988.

22. Delmez JA: Peripheral nerve entrapment syndromes in chronic hemodialysis patients. *Nephron* 30:118–123, 1982.

23. Katz SG, Kohl RD: The percutaneous treatment of angioaccess graft complications. *Am J Surg* 170:238–242, 1995.

24. Kumpe DA, Cohen MA: Angioplasty/thrombolytic treatment of failing and failed hemodialysis access sites: Comparison with surgical treatment. *Prog Cardiovasc Dis* 34:263–278, 1992.
25. Shoenfeld R, Hermans H, Novick A, et al: Stenting of proximal venous obstructions to maintain hemodialysis access. *J Vasc Surg* 19:532–539, 1994.
26. Beathard GA: Thrombolysis versus surgery for the treatment of thrombosed dialysis access grafts. *J Am Soc Nephrol* 6:1619–1624, 1995.

PART V

Aortic Disease

CHAPTER 6

Critical Pathways for Abdominal Aortic Aneurysms*

Keith D. Calligaro, M.D.
Section of Vascular Surgery, Pennsylvania Hospital/University of Pennsylvania School of Medicine, Philadelphia, Pennsylvania

Rahul Dandura
Section of Vascular Surgery, Pennsylvania Hospital/University of Pennsylvania School of Medicine, Philadelphia, Pennsylvania

Matthew J. Dougherty, M.D.
Section of Vascular Surgery, Pennsylvania Hospital/University of Pennsylvania School of Medicine, Philadelphia, Pennsylvania

Carol A. Raviola, M.D.
Section of Vascular Surgery, Pennsylvania Hospital/University of Pennsylvania School of Medicine, Philadelphia, Pennsylvania

Dominic A. DeLaurentis, M.D.
Section of Vascular Surgery, Pennsylvania Hospital/University of Pennsylvania School of Medicine, Philadelphia, Pennsylvania

I n this era of managed health care, critical (or clinical) pathways have been established as a means of decreasing health care costs while simultaneously increasing efficiency and possibly decreasing adverse outcomes of major surgery. Implementation of these pathways is essential for vascular surgeons. In the future, resource utilization, cost-effectiveness, and outcome may be quantified for various types of operations and reflect on the competence and efficiency of individual surgeons.[1-3] In addition to minimizing costs, critical pathways have also been shown to diminish adverse out-

*Supported by a grant from the John F. Connelly Foundation and the Pennsylvania Hospital Funds.

Advances in Vascular Surgery®, vol. 5
©1997, Mosby–Year Book, Inc.

comes through the development of practice standards and guide-lines.[4] We previously reported methods that we used to decrease hospital costs for patients who underwent carotid, aortic, and lower-extremity vascular surgery[4] and, more specifically, surgery for aortoiliac aneurysms and occlusive disease.[5] In this chapter, we will detail the critical pathway that we established for patients undergoing elective abdominal aortic aneurysm (AAA) surgery and the consequences of pathway implementation.

PATIENTS AND METHODS

Before a critical pathway was adopted for AAA surgery in early 1994, patients were routinely admitted at least 1 day before surgery for a variety of reasons. All or most preoperative testing, including laboratory and radiologic studies, were performed on an inpatient basis. Arteriography was usually performed in the inpatient setting the day before surgery. This avoided the inconvenience to the patient of multiple hospital visits. Consulting physicians evaluated the patient during this preoperative hospital stay. Any necessary cardiac, pulmonary, or other tests were obtained, which not infrequently resulted in the postponement of surgery, such as when tests could not be performed in a prompt fashion or when test results prompted further investigation. Even in the rare instance when all these preoperative evaluations were completed before admission for surgery, we favored admission the day before surgery for overnight IV hydration and bowel preparation. The primary reasons for our prior approach were patient and physician convenience, but we also believed that this strategy was the safest for patients undergoing such major operations.

In early 1994, we implemented a critical pathway for patients undergoing elective AAA surgery at Pennsylvania Hospital. This change in strategy was a result of prompting by our hospital administration, who believed that attaining shorter length of hospital stays and decreasing hospital costs were essential to remaining competitive in the overcrowded health care system in our area. All vascular surgeons at our hospital and representatives of our hospital administration, nursing, and anesthesia departments met with a team of health care consultants on a monthly basis during a 1-year period. These advisors demonstrated the urgent need to establish critical pathways for all types of vascular surgery to decrease costs, optimally without adversely affecting our low morbidity and mortality rates. In addition, the vascular surgeons frequently met with a vascular nurse coordinator to decide on uniform, specific preoperative and postoperative algorithms. Obtaining a consensus on such matters as when to remove nasogastric tubes and Foley and epidural catheters and when to obtain postoperative hemoglobin levels and chest radiographs was often associated with vigorous and lively discussion.

As a direct consequence of these meetings, we changed two specific operative factors associated with repair of AAAs. We agreed that epidural catheters would be inserted and left in place until the third postoperative day for all patients. It has been our impression that use of epidural analgesia greatly helped patients ambulate sooner and improved respiratory mechanics because of lessened incisional pain. We also began to perform AAA surgery preferentially through a retroperitoneal approach when involvement of the right iliac artery was limited. It was our belief, supported by others, that this incision is associated with less pain, better respiratory function, and fewer intestinal motility problems than a midline incision.[6, 7] If the aneurysm extended far onto the right common iliac artery, we repaired the aneurysm through a midline approach.

We initially agreed on three overall changes in strategy. First, all preoperative assessment was performed in an outpatient setting. Second, patients were admitted the morning of surgery. Third, early discharge was planned via the establishment of routine, preprinted postoperative orders. Preoperative assessment was performed on an outpatient basis and included all laboratory and radiologic studies, as well as arteriography. Cardiology and anesthesiology evaluations were also performed before admission. Where possible, this and other preoperative testing was performed in conjunction with outpatient arteriography. Although we continue to perform arteriography before all elective aortic aneurysm surgery, other vascular surgeons omit this diagnostic procedure and are instead willing to operate with US or CT evaluations only. Both these tests are less expensive and less hazardous than arteriography, which may be reserved for juxtarenal or suprarenal aneurysms. Still others prefer CT angiography as an alternative method to evaluate aortic aneurysms. Partial bowel preparation consisted of a clear liquid diet and a Fleet enema the day before surgery. However, preoperative evaluations could not be routinely performed in 1 day on all patients. Because many patients lived more than an hour away, they needed to be inconvenienced to a great degree. An example of our preoperative checklist is included as Table 1.

The morning of surgery, patients are brought to a holding area immediately adjacent to the operating room for the placement of

TABLE 1.

Preoperative Checklist for Elective Infrarenal Abdominal
Aortic Aneurysms

Consultations as necessary
Consent
History and physical examination
Diet: clear liquids the day before surgery, with nothing by mouth the
  morning of surgery
Fleet enema the night before surgery
Laboratory tests: complete blood count, prothrombin time/partial
  thromboplastin time, SMA-7, urinalysis, type and crossmatch of 4 U of
  peripheral red blood cells
Electrocardiogram
Chest radiograph

IV lines and final anesthesiology evaluation. Pulmonary artery
catheters are inserted in the operating room before induction of anesthesia. Patients traveling long distances are encouraged to use
discounted local hotels the night before surgery. This strategy was
also implemented by our hospital administration.

Postoperative order forms that the vascular surgeons had previously agreed on were reviewed and cosigned by the surgical
housestaff. These orders included diet (nothing by mouth until
clear liquids the second or third postoperative day and advancement to a regular diet on the fourth or fifth day), laboratory tests
(hemoglobin, electrolytes, blood urea nitrogen, and creatinine in
the recovery room and then only the first postoperative morning
unless the clinical situation dictated otherwise; on the second postoperative morning only electrolytes), radiologic studies (chest radiograph in the recovery room and not repeated the next morning
unless clinically indicated), ambulation (out of bed in a chair the
first postoperative day and ambulating with assistance the second
day), and physical therapy consultations only when absolutely necessary (as another means of decreasing costs) (Table 2). Our goal
was to transfer patients from the ICU to a designated vascular ward
on the first postoperative day if they were hemodynamically stable
and no other significant medical concerns existed. Discharge was
planned for the fifth postoperative day after AAA surgery.

We compared morbidity, mortality, length of hospital stay, and
hospital costs among 85 patients admitted for elective AAA before

(group I, 47 patients) and after implementation of the critical pathways (group II, 38 patients) between July 1, 1992, and December 31, 1995, to the vascular service at Pennsylvania Hospital in Philadelphia. Patients who underwent AAA surgery during this time were excluded from analysis if they required admission before the day of surgery to optimize their medical status (e.g., IV hydration

---

TABLE 2.
Postoperative Orders for Elective Infrarenal Abdominal Aortic
Aneurysm Surgery

On arrival at the recovery room:
  Laboratory tests: SMA-7, hemoglobin and hematocrit, platelet count,
    arterial blood gas, ECG, chest radiograph
  Vital signs per ICU protocol
  Triflow and chest physical therapy every hour
  Nasogastric tube to low intermittent suction
  Antithrombotic pumps
  Monitor arterial line, pulmonary artery catheter, pulse oximetry
  Call house officer if temperature is greater than 101.5°F, blood
    pressure is greater than 170 or less than 110 mm Hg systolic, heart
    rate is greater than 120 or less than 50 beats/min, urine output is
    less than 60 mL/2 hr
  Pain medications per epidural catheter
  Sucralfate per nasogastric tube
Postoperative date 1:
  4 A.M.: SMA-7, complete blood count, platelet count, ECG
  Out of bed in chair before transfer
  Remove nasogastric tube, arterial line, pulmonary artery catheter
  Transfer to vascular ward
Postoperative day 2:
  6:00 A.M.: hemoglobin and hematocrit, electrolytes
  Out of bed—ambulate 3 times per day
Postoperative day 3:
  Discontinue epidural catheter
  Clear liquids by mouth
Postoperative day 4:
  Convert IV to heparin lock
  Regular diet
Postoperative day 5:
  Discharge

in preparation for renal surgery, optimization of cardiac function, prolonged preoperative antibiotics) or if they could not undergo preoperative testing on an elective outpatient basis (e.g., emergency surgery, transfers from another service or hospital).

Cost analysis for patients undergoing AAA surgery was based on patient billing. The analysis was performed during the initial baseline period and at the final tracking period. Health care consultants retained by the hospital administration applied a variable cost ratio of the cost to charges supplied by the hospital. Annual cost savings refer only to the hospital setting, and costs in the outpatient setting were not included.

RESULTS

No significant differences ($P > 0.05$) were noted between groups I and II in age, sex, race, diabetes mellitus, hypertension, hypercholesterolemia, pulmonary disease, cardiac disease, preoperative cardiac testing, renal insufficiency, or insertion of intraoperative pulmonary artery catheters. Significantly more group II patients had surgery performed via a retroperitoneal approach (60% [23/38] vs. 17% [8/47], $P = 0.001$) and had epidural analgesia (91% [35/38] vs. 65% [31/47], $P = 0.001$) than did group I patients.

Despite same-day admissions and other cost-saving strategies, no significant differences were found between groups I and II in terms of mortality (0%); cardiac (2.1% [1/47] vs. 0%), pulmonary (10% [5/47] vs. 5% [2/38]), or renal (2.1% [1/47] vs. 0%) complications; or readmission rates within 30 days (4.2% [2/47] vs. 5.3% [2/38], respectively, $P > 0.05$). The one cardiac complication consisted of pulmonary edema and ventricular arrythmias in a group I patient. The 7 pulmonary complications included 4 patients in whom pneumonia developed and 3 who required reintubation or prolonged intubation (> 48 hours postoperatively) for respiratory insufficiency. In 1 patient in group I, a permanent elevation in serum creatinine developed after undergoing repair of an aortic aneurysm and a left renal bypass, but this patient did not require dialysis. Two patients in group I were readmitted within 30 days of discharge (atrial fibrillation, small-bowel obstruction), as well as 3 patients in group II (2 incisional hernias, 1 deep vein thrombosis).

There were significant decreases in length of hospital stay (6 vs. 11 days, $P < 0.0001$) as a result of decreased preoperative and postoperative stay, length of stay in the ICU (1.2 vs. 2.3 days, $P < 0.0001$), and hospital cost per patient ($34,000 vs. $45,000, $P = 0.001$) for group II patients as compared with group I.

DISCUSSION

This study demonstrated that the majority of patients requiring elective AAA surgery at our hospital could be admitted the day of surgery and undergo early discharge with significant hospital cost savings and without an apparent increase in morbidity or mortality. Before the recent focus on cost containment, patients who required aortic surgery were routinely admitted to our hospital before the day of surgery for medical evaluation, arteriography, IV hydration, and the convenience of both the physician and patient. We and others have previously reported the safety and efficacy of same-day admissions for carotid and lower-extremity bypasses.[4-6, 8, 9] The results of the current study clearly show that admission before the day of surgery is also not necessary for the majority of patients undergoing elective AAA surgery.

However, several factors should be emphasized. Implementation of clinical pathways proved to be a time-consuming endeavor on the part of the physicians and hospital administration. As previously detailed, a team of professional health care advisors met with the vascular surgeons, senior administration officials, and nursing, cardiology, and anesthesiology representatives over a lengthy period to decide which strategies were cost-effective and practical. Clinical protocols were reviewed in detail and agreed on by the vascular surgeons. This required the establishment of consensus and willingness to confront and eliminate personal biases through group discussion. Establishment of a dedicated vascular wing of the hospital was essential to guarantee standards of nursing care. Likewise, education and involvement of surgical residents and the vascular fellow were crucial to success.

Although significant hospital cost savings were realized, physicians had to meet the need for more nursing and secretarial personnel in the office to handle increased outpatient test scheduling, patient education, and insurance details. Earlier discharge led to more frequent postoperative physician office visits. Costs were also shifted to outpatient nursing and physical therapy because many patients required these services as a result of earlier discharge. This approach also led to more inconvenience and expenses on the part of the patients and their families, although with adequate education and management of expectations there were few complaints. Our hospital is a tertiary referral center, and many patients need to travel 1 or 2 hours. Many patients who did not stay in a nearby hotel but instead came to the hospital the morning of surgery needed to awaken at 3:00 A.M., leave their homes by

4:00 A.M., and travel 2 hours to arrive in registration by 6:00 A.M. and undergo the previously mentioned preparations. Understandably, a few patients absolutely insisted that they be admitted the day before surgery. If their insurance company made this allowance (which has become very rare), we would accommodate the patient. It should be noted that we did not encounter one patient who was willing to pay the hospital bill out of his own pocket for a preoperative overnight stay if the insurance company did not cover this cost. It should also be realized that a few patients who traveled far distances during their repeated preoperative testing or on the morning of surgery complained frequently and vehemently to their surgeon about these inconveniences.

Approximately 20% of the patients who required AAA surgery at our hospital during the study period were not candidates for clinical pathways. This proportion will vary among different hospitals depending on the number of patients who require emergency surgery and the prevalence of significant medical risk factors. Tertiary care hospitals such as ours that accept complicated, high-risk patients transferred from other hospitals will necessarily have more patients excluded from portions of the protocol, although cost savings can still be realized to a lesser extent and the overall philosophy remains consistent.

This study did not identify any significant differences in medical risk factors between the two groups of patients. However, because patients who were admitted before the day of surgery to optimize their medical status were excluded from analysis, some bias may have been introduced in this retrospective review.

As previously mentioned, we changed our strategy in performing AAA surgery as a result of implementing clinical pathways through the routine use of epidural analgesia and preferential use of a retroperitoneal approach. We analyzed whether these factors may also have resulted in earlier discharge for group II patients. With regard to the latter, a retroperitoneal approach for aortic surgery has been reported to result in shorter hospital stays,[6] although others have not confirmed this finding.[10] Although we performed these operations through a retroperitoneal approach more frequently in group II patients, our previously reported findings on this subject showed no significant difference in the length of hospital stay for group II patients whether the operation was performed with this approach or via a midline incision.[5] Our results demonstrate that implementation of clinical pathways and changes in physicians' attitudes may play a more important role in decreasing the length of hospital stay and hospital costs than might the type of incision.

The other perioperative factor that differed between the two groups was that significantly more patients in group II than group I had epidural analgesia. This change in strategy was a result of implementing clinical pathways after discussions with our anesthesiologists. The potential advantages of epidural analgesia for patients undergoing AAA surgery are less postoperative pain, earlier ambulation, and earlier discharge.[7, 11] However, very few group II patients had general anesthesia without epidural analgesia, so a valid analysis of this factor as it related to length of hospital stay was not possible.

CONCLUSION

Our results demonstrate that the majority of patients undergoing elective AAA surgery can be admitted the morning of surgery and discharged from the hospital in an expeditious manner without adversely affecting outcome. It is clear that increased efforts, inconvenience, and cost on the part of both the patient and surgeon will be required to meet challenges in the current health care environment.

REFERENCES

1. Wilmore DW: Enhancing surgical competence during rapid changes in health care delivery. *Ann Surg* 221:supplement, 1995.
2. Graham RG, DePorter JG: An approach to assessing resource utilization and clinical outcomes in a hospital setting. *Top Health Care Finance* 18:53–57, 1991.
3. Deterling RA Jr: Presidential address: Quality assurance and medical economics—their impact on the practice of surgery. *J Vasc Surg* 12:640–644, 1990.
4. Calligaro KD, Dougherty MJ, Raviola CA, et al: Impact of clinical pathways on hospital costs and early outcome after major vascular surgery. *J Vasc Surg* 22:649–660, 1995.
5. Calligaro KD, Dandura R, Dougherty MJ, et al: Same-day admissions and other cost saving strategies for elective aortoiliac surgery. *J Vasc Surg* 25:41–44, 1997.
6. Sicard GA, Reilly JM, Rubin BG, et al: Transabdominal versus retroperitoneal incision for abdominal aortic surgery: Report of a prospective randomized trial. *J Vasc Surg* 21:174–181, 1995.
7. Rosenbaum GJ, Arroyo PJ, Sivina M: Retroperitoneal approach used exclusively with epidural anesthesia for infrarenal aortic disease. *Am J Surg* 168:136–139, 1994.
8. Collier PE: Carotid endarterectomy: A safe and cost-efficient approach. *J Vasc Surg* 16:926–933, 1992.
9. Musser DJ, Calligaro KD, Dougherty MJ, et al: Safety and cost-efficiency of 24-hour hospitalization for carotid endarterectomy. *Ann Vasc Surg* 10:143–146, 1996.

10. Cambria RP, Brewster DC, Abbott WM, et al: Transperitoneal versus retroperitoneal approach for aortic reconstruction: A randomized prospective study. *J Vasc Surg* 11:314–325, 1990.

11. Katz, S, Reiten P, Kohl R: The use of epidural anaesthesia and analgesia in aortic surgery. *Am Surg* 58:470–473, 1992.

CHAPTER 7

Epidural Cooling for the Prevention of Spinal Cord Ischemic Complications After Thoracoabdominal Aortic Surgery

Richard P. Cambria, M.D.

Associate Professor of Surgery, Harvard Medical School, Boston, Massachusetts; Visiting Surgeon, Department of Vascular Surgery, Massachusetts General Hospital, Boston, Massachusetts

J. Kenneth Davison, D.D.S., M.D.

Associate Professor of Anesthesia, Harvard Medical School, Boston Massachusetts; Anesthetist, Department of Anesthesia, Massachusetts General Hospital, Boston, Massachusetts

A variety of surgical and nonsurgical adjuncts notwithstanding, spinal cord ischemia remains an unsolved problem in surgical resection of the thoracic and thoracoabdominal aorta. Earlier problems, specifically, extensive perioperative hemorrhage and clinically significant renal failure, occur infrequently after elective operations in contemporary practice. Perhaps the best barometer of the overall risk of cord injury emanates from Crawford's monumental experience with over 1,500 patients wherein a 16% overall risk of lower-extremity neurologic deficit was reported; half of these complications resulted in devastatingly complete paraplegia, disallowing any meaningful rehabilitation.[1] Alternatively, most patients with milder forms of injury (i.e., paraparesis) will recover sufficiently with rehabilitation to be independently ambulatory. Therefore, seeking to limit the overall extent of cord injury is a worthwhile goal.

Although Crawford's data must be considered the benchmark because of their sheer magnitude, a variety of contemporary reports suggest that the overall incidence of spinal cord injury may be significantly less than that suggested from the original Baylor experience.[2-8] Indeed, those who have carried on Dr. Crawford's work have reported overall rates of spinal cord ischemic complications in the 5% to 7% range,[4,5] figures consistent with our own experience.[6-8] Despite this, few would suggest that cord ischemia is a solved problem, and because the consequences of paraplegia are devastating, substantial investigative efforts have been devoted to its prevention. There is general consensus that a variety of clinical variables strongly influence the overall risk of spinal cord injury during the course of thoracoabdominal aortic aneurysm (TAA) resection. These variables include the duration of aortic cross-clamping, aneurysm extent, emergency operations, and chronic dissection, although the latter has recently been disputed.[5] Acher et al. incorporated most of these variables into the formulation of a predictive model for neurologic deficit after TAA repair. They demonstrated excellent correlation ($r = 0.997$) between the predicted incidence of neurologic deficits from their model and that actually reported in 16 published series.[2] Crawford et al. demonstrated that for each extent of TAA, risk of cord injury increased with increased duration of aortic clamping. Paraplegia was rare when clamp duration was less than 30 minutes but rose dramatically when the ischemic period was longer than 60 minutes.[1] Experience in our unit has verified the importance of cross-clamp duration. When we examined the impact of epidural cooling on ischemic cord complications, we noted in 125 patients with types I, II, and III TAA that a visceral cross-clamp time longer than 60 minutes was associated with ischemic cord injury ($P = 0.02$).[7] In the authors' personal series of 160 patients treated over the past decade, surgery for ruptured TAA has been the single most impressive correlate ($P = 0.001$) of postoperative spinal cord complications.[8]

There is considerable divergence of opinion and practice with respect to the operative management of TAA, and much of this is driven by varying perspectives on the optimal method(s) to prevent cord injury. Clinical strategies to decrease the risk of ischemic cord complications can be divided into two general categories (Table 1). The first of these categories consists of maneuvers designed to identify, preserve, or maintain critical spinal cord blood supply. These maneuvers include preoperative angiographic localization of critical intercostal vessels,[9,10] intraoperative identification of the same vessels with either the H_2 ion electrode method[11] or evoked potential monitoring,[12] the use of shunts/bypasses for

TABLE 1.
Strategies to Prevent Spinal Cord Ischemia During
Thoracoabdominal Aortic Aneurysm Repair

Maintenance of spinal cord blood supply
  Identification of critical segmental (intercostal) vessels
    Preoperative selective angiography
    Intraoperative H_2 ion method
    Intraoperative evoked potential monitoring
  Shunts and bypasses—distal aortic perfusion
    Passive internal (Gott) or external (axillofemoral) shunt
    Atriofemoral or femoral-femoral bypass (partial CP bypass)
    Complete CP Bypass (with/without circulatory arrest/profound
    hypothermia)
  CSF Drainage
  Intercostal/lumbar vessel reanastomosis
  Intrathecal vasodilators
Neuroprotective adjuncts
  Hypothermia
    Systemic
      Passive (moderate)
      Active (moderate or profound—with CP bypass)
    Regional (moderate)
      Epidural or intrathecal infusion (closed or drained)
      Isolated aortic segment perfusion
  Pharmacologic agents
    Neurotransmitter inhibition (naloxone)
    Nonspecific neuroprotective agents (steroids, barbiturates)
    Calcium channel blockers
    Oxygen free radical scavengers
    Artificial O_2 delivery (Fluosol-DA)

Abbreviations: CP, cardiopulmonary; *DA,* delayed action.

distal aortic perfusion,[4, 5] CSF drainage,[4, 13] and intercostal vessel reanastomosis.[14] Frequently, combinations of these techniques are applied. The second general category involves so-called neuroprotective adjuncts whose use is specifically intended to increase ischemic tolerance of the spinal cord, especially during the cross-clamp interval. These adjuncts include hypothermia, either regional (on the cord itself) or systemic, and a variety of pharmacologic agents. Several classifications of pharmacologic agents based on their respective mechanisms of action can be used: nonspecific neuroprotective agents, e.g., steroids, prostaglandins, and barbiturates; excitatory neurotransmitter inhibitors, e.g., naloxone; and calcium channel blockers and O_2 free radical scavengers, both of which act at different points on the cascade of reperfusion injury.

In the clinical setting it may be difficult or impossible to differentiate the benefit of any one modality because they are often used in combination. It is not the purpose of the present review to consider all of these strategies, which have been reviewed elsewhere.[15, 16] Herein we develop a rationale for the use of regional hypothermia for spinal cord protection based on fundamental considerations of spinal cord blood supply and the pathogenesis of cord injury relevant to patients with TAA.

REVIEW OF SPINAL CORD BLOOD SUPPLY

Even in the nonpathologic state, human spinal cord circulation is extremely variable, and "normal" anatomy is frequently altered by mural thrombus or dissection in an aneurysm. There may be great variability in the principal and collateral circulation that any individual patient brings to the clinical setting. Therefore, even among patients with equivalent aneurysm extent, the risk of ischemic spinal cord damage may vary greatly.

The circulation to the cord can be divided into two interconnected parts: the intrinsic and the extrinsic circulation (Fig 1,A). The intrinsic circulation is composed of a single anterior and paired posterior spinal arteries that travel in the anterior median sulcus and on the posterior columns, respectively. The most important branches are the perforating central arteries from the anterior spinal artery, which supply 75% of the spinal cord substance.

The extrinsic circulation includes the radicular and medullary arteries and can be considered the feeders of the intrinsic circulation. Radicular arteries travel with the nerve roots and may or may not continue on as medullary arteries that ultimately contribute to the intrinsic circulation. The principal extrinsic blood supply in the cervical and upper thoracic region is provided by the vertebral arteries. The thoracolumbar cord is supplied by the intercostal and lumbar arteries, and the conus is supplied by the lateral sacral branches of the hypogastric vessels. It is not commonly appreciated that very few of these segmental aortic branches directly contribute to the intrinsic circulation of the spinal cord. For example, posterior branches of the intercostal arteries do contribute radicular arteries at many levels, but most of these supply only the nerve

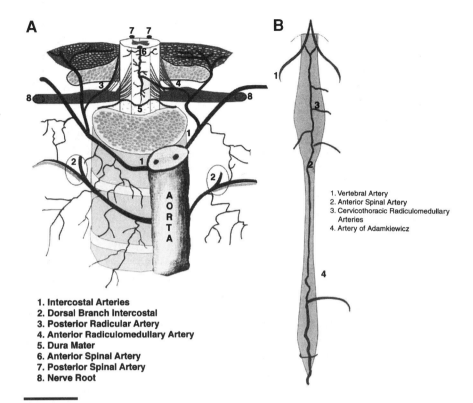

A, schematic of the extrinsic and intrinsic circulation of the human spinal cord.

1. Intercostal Arteries
2. Dorsal Branch Intercostal
3. Posterior Radicular Artery
4. Anterior Radiculomedullary Artery
5. Dura Mater
6. Anterior Spinal Artery
7. Posterior Spinal Artery
8. Nerve Root

1. Vertebral Artery
2. Anterior Spinal Artery
3. Cervicothoracic Radiculomedullary Arteries
4. Artery of Adamkiewicz

FIGURE 1.

A, schematic of the extrinsic and intrinsic circulation of the human spinal cord. Note that the posterior branch of left intercostal does contribute the medullary artery in this representation. **B,** course and relative caliber changes of the anterior spinal artery *(ASA)* and its anastomotic connection with the artery of Adamkiewicz *(GRA)*. Note the narrow caliber of the ASA cephalad to the entry point of the GRA. (Adapted from Schepens MA: *The Surgical Treatment of Thoracoabdominal Aortic Aneurysms.* Unpublished doctoral dissertation.)

roots and do not actually contribute to a medullary (actually reaching the cord substance) artery. Therefore, the circulation of any particular region of the cord will vary depending on how many radicular arteries actually contribute medullary components. In fact, only a total of seven or eight radiculomedullary arteries supply the entire intrinsic circulation of the human spinal cord.

An additional important concept to appreciate is the variability in both size and continuity of the anterior spinal artery. Although it is true that this is largely a continuous vessel traveling in the central sulcus, the vessel itself becomes extremely narrow in the middle thoracic region and often shows one or more breaks in continuity (Fig 1,B). The peculiarities of anatomy of the anterior spinal artery explain why the richly perfused cervical anterior spinal artery (which rises from branches of the vertebral artery) may not be adequate to sustain viability of the cord should the more caudal radiculomedullary feeder arteries be interrupted. Thus, the human spinal cord has several functionally isolated vascular territories that are potentially ischemic if the radiculomedullary vessels are interrupted. The three main anatomical and functionally isolated vascular territories are the upper cervicothoracic territory, the intermediate thoracic territory from approximately T4 to T8, and the lower thoracolumbar territory from T9 to the conus medullaris. The cervicothoracic territory has a rich potential collateral circulation, and ischemic injury in this region is distinctly uncommon under any circumstance. The principal segmental spinal arteries in this region arise mainly from the vertebral arteries, and this short segment has at least four genuine radiculomedullary arteries. Although the middle thoracic segment appears to have but one or two radiculomedullary arteries, the anterior spinal artery in this region continues to be well developed. Experienced surgeons will recognize that with a proximal descending thoracic aortic clamp, the intercostal artery orifices in the T4 to T8 region are generally vigorously backbleeding when the aorta is opened, which is indicative of adequate collateral circulation to the potential segmental feeder vessels from this region of the upper thoracic aorta. Alternatively, the thoracolumbar territory is at greatest risk for ischemic injury because this region is mostly supplied by a single radiculomedullary artery. This largest radiculomedullary artery, which is critical to the circulation of the thoracolumbar cord, was originally described in 1882 by Adamkiewicz. It is commonly referred to as the arteria radicularis magna (ARM), the great radiculomedullary artery, or alternatively the artery of Adamkiewicz. The anterior spinal artery just cephalad to the anastomotic point of the ARM is extremely small, whereas just caudal to the entry of the ARM it is relatively wide (see Fig 1). The ARM enters the vertebral canal between the 9th and 12th thoracic vertebral segments 75% of the time. Angiographic studies have shown that one or more intercostal arteries can contribute to the ARM.[9, 10] Because of variability in the level of origin in the thoracolumbar segment and the vagaries of contributions to the ARM from multiple potential intercostal vessels, one strategy to limit ischemic complications has been attempts to precisely depict the anatomy of the ARM with preoperative angiographic studies. Kieffer et al. demonstrated that the risk of neurologic deficit is highest when the aortic segment from which critical intercostal vessels arise needs to be encompassed in the resection.[10] Savader et al. reported that the ARM could be identified by specific preoperative spinal arteriography in 65% of the patients in whom this technique was attempted. Their angiographic studies were consistent with prior anatomical studies with respect to the level of origin of the ARM. In 78% of the patients studied, the ARM originated between the T9 and T12 levels, and in most of these patients, the arteries ultimately supplying the ARM were left intercostals. These authors also confirmed that the anterior spinal artery may be discontinuous thus reinforcing the fact that the thoracolumbar segment may be entirely dependent on its segmental radiculomedullary blood supply (i.e., emphasizing the importance of the ARM). Unfortunately, clinical benefit from accurate preoperative localization of the critical intercostals that contribute to the ARM could not be demonstrated. Overall morbidity and mortality, including spinal cord ischemic injury, were no different in those patients in whom the critical intercostals could be identified as opposed to those in whom it could not. However, consistent with the Kieffer data, in patients in whom the critical intercostals were not included in the aneurysm resection, a zero incidence of neurologic morbidity was noted as compared with 50% in those whose resection involved the critical aortic segment.[9]

PATHOGENESIS OF ISCHEMIC INJURY TO THE SPINAL CORD

In the presence of a proximal descending aortic clamp, spinal cord perfusion will depend on the caliber and continuity of the anterior spinal artery, the presence of patent critical intercostal vessels distal to the clamp, and the difference between arterial pressure in the spinal arteries and CSF pressure. The latter has been referred to as the relative spinal cord perfusion pressure, a concept developed to illustrate the potential negative impact of increased CSF pressure on cord perfusion. However, the assumption that spinal arterial pressure equals distal (below the clamp) aortic pressure is probably incorrect.[17, 18] Proximal thoracic aortic clamping can result in increased CSF pressure thought to be secondary to the abrupt increase in cranial blood flow. Our experience has been that this response in patients is variable; although elevated CSF pressure can be seen in very proximal arch clamping, the majority of patients exhibit modest changes in CSF pressure with clamping. Furthermore, experimental evidence indicates that elevated CSF pressure compromises spinal cord blood flow only when CSF pressure is artifactually elevated to at least four times baseline values.[19]

Ultimately, cord injury after aortic replacement results from an ischemic insult that can be in the form of either temporary interruption (during clamping) or permanent sacrifice of the principal or collateral extrinsic cord blood supply. However, there continues to be debate about the relative importance of the initial ischemic insult and the secondary reperfusion or hyperemic phase that can cause cord swelling and become clinically evident hours to days after the operative procedure. An understanding of the progression of events that can lead to clinical cord injury continues to be driven by the fact that up to 50% of neurologic deficits in some series have been observed to occur hours, days, or even weeks postoperatively. Individual case reports of dramatic reversal of neurologic deficits with such maneuvers as the administration of naloxone[2] or CSF drainage[20] have been noted.

More importantly, the fluctuation or occurrence of neurologic deficits seen hours or days after surgery often correlate with hemodynamic instability. Svenssen et al. reported that 50% of the neurologic deficits in a series of 100 carefully studied patients occurred in a delayed fashion, and their manuscript reveals a 30% incidence of postoperative hypotension.[14] We have observed examples of this, particularly in the setting of postoperative bleeding or hemodynamic instability during hemodialysis. These observations strongly suggest that the blood supply to the cord is in a fragile balance for days to weeks after surgery, and every effort should be made to maintain adequate perfusion pressure in the days after TAA aortic resection. Other mechanisms such as thrombosis of reconstructed intercostal arteries and microembolization may contribute to the development of delayed deficits.

On a cellular level, many components of neuronal injury and death are similar to the pathophysiology of other ischemic tissues, with the important exception that neural tissue is more sensitive to ischemic insults. Similar to intracellular processes affecting ischemic tissue in general, ischemic neurons accumulate abnormal levels of intracellular calcium, which has been implicated in the release of neurotoxic excitatory neurotransmitters such as glutamate. Microsphere studies have demonstrated that a hyperemic response occurs in the cord after a period of clamp-induced ischemia. There is evidence that hypothermia blunts this hyperemic response. Similar to the reperfusion phenomenon in other tissues, free radical generation occurs in the presence of the enzyme xanthine oxidase. The principal cellular toxic effect of free radicals relates to lipid peroxidation with the resultant loss of membrane-dependent enzyme systems and a consequent inability of the cell to regulate its internal environment. Many pharmacologic adjuncts directed toward components of reperfusion injury have been evaluated with inconsistent results in experimental systems and with scant clinical data.

INTERCOSTAL VESSEL SACRIFICE OR REANASTOMOSIS?

Sacrifice of critical intercostal vessels that supply the ARM and the inability to reperfuse these arteries in a *timely* fashion are acknowledged by most to be central to the pathogenesis of ischemic cord injury. From a practical standpoint, reanastomosis of intercostal vessels can be technically difficult or even impossible in circumstances in which excessive atheroma or an acute dissection surrounds the intercostal ostia. Furthermore, even with attempts at reanastomosis by the inclusion button method, postoperative angiographic studies have suggested that these reconstructions may fail in a significant percentage of patients. Although we have not routinely performed postoperative angiograms, we have had the opportunity to observe patent postoperative intercostal vessel reconstructions in many patients when studied by postoperative arteriography. It is the authors' opinion that there is now sufficient angiographic evidence in humans indicating that the ARM originates between T8 and L1 in nearly all patients and that attempts at intercostal vessel reanastomosis should be directed toward this region. An indication of the collateralization or lack thereof to these vessels is commonly observed in the operating room when an extensive thoracoabdominal aneurysm is opened. Typically, with a clamp just distal to the subclavian, intercostal vessels between T4 and T8 are vigorously backbleeding and can be an important source of blood loss. It is our practice to routinely oversew vessels in this region as quickly as possible and to balloon-occlude those vessels in the critical zone selected for subsequent reconstruction.

The studies of Wadouh et al.[17] and Dapunt et al.[18] give credence to the theory that freely backbleeding or intercostal vessels exposed only to atmospheric pressure can create a steal phenomenon and actually decrease relative spinal cord perfusion. It must be acknowledged, however, that intercostal vessel reanastomosis is usually a "blind" maneuver unless some method of preoperative or intraoperative localization of the critical intercostal vessels is applied. Acher et al. suggested that expending aortic clamp time for intercostal vessel reanastomosis was a worthless maneuver, and they routinely oversewed all intercostal vessels with the adjunctive use of CSF drainage and IV naloxone and reported an overall neurologic deficit rate of 3% in 56 patients.[2] However, these authors must be considered in the minority, and most agree that sacrifice of the critical intercostal vessels is the single most important factor in the development of postoperative spinal cord injury and therefore believe that such vessels should be reanastomosed.

Svenssen et al. reported the most detailed study of a specific level of intercostal vessel management available.[14] These investigators prospectively mapped the number and level of patent intercostal vessels and whether such vessels were reattached. They reported a 32% rate of overall spinal cord injury, half of which were devastating paraplegia. Patients who had sacrifice of patent intercostal vessels at the T8 to L1 level had a much higher incidence of spinal cord injury than did those who did not have sacrifice of vessels at this level. There was a statistically significant improvement in the neurologic injury rate for those patients who had reanastomosis of vessels in this critical region when compared with those who did not. Although these investigators concluded that intercostal reanastomosis at this level was an important adjunct, an equally valid conclusion would be that intercostal vessel reanastomosis *alone* was insufficient to prevent cord injury because there was still a 30% deficit rate in patients who underwent reconstruction of vessels in the critical zone. We believe that such intercostal reanastomosis may be inadequate simply because it cannot be performed quickly enough, hence the rationale for hypothermic cord protection during the cross-clamp interval.

Indirect but compelling evidence for the spinal cord's narrow "ischemic window" is available from contemporary studies using direct spinal cord somatosensory evoked potential (scSSEP) monitoring. This technique provides for direct epidural electrode stimulation and recording of potentials from the posterior columns of the cord itself. The largest clinical series with scSSEP was reported by Grabitz et al., who used two electrodes placed directly in the epidural space, one at the L1–2 level for stimulation and one at the T5–6 level for recording.[12] This system proved to be safe and technically successful in 167 of the 172 patients (97%) in whom it was attempted. Eighty percent of their patients had types I, II, or III TAA (i.e., likely to have resection of the critical aortic segment), and bypass and distal perfusion techniques were not used. The authors observed a range of response in the scSSEP after aortic clamping. Approximately one third of their patients had no diminution in scSSEP after aortic clamping, and there were no neurologic deficits in this group. Presumably, these patients have either well-developed anterior spinal arteries or established collateral circulation not dependent on aortic branches distal to the clamp. Another third of their patients experienced an intermediate response with initially normal scSSEPs, which began to dissipate 15 minutes after placement of the aortic clamp. Overall, neurologic deficits occurred in 16% in this group. In the group of patients who experienced rapid (within 15 minutes of aortic clamping) loss of scSSEPs, the neurologic deficit rate was 26%. The overall rate of lower-extremity neurologic deficit in the entire series was 15%, with the ratio of paraparesis to paraplegia running 2:1.

Not surprisingly, absence of scSSEP loss after aortic clamping varied with the extent of aneurysm; 75% of the patients with type IV aneurysm had no change in potentials with clamping. However, only 25% of the patients with the more extensive type I and type II aneurysms had no loss of scSSEPs with clamping. The most severe type of response, i.e., loss of potentials in less than 15 minutes, was seen in at least one third of the patients with type I, II, and III aneurysms. Neurologic outcome for each group of SSEP response was correlated with the ability to achieve *rapid* return of scSSEP with early intercostal vessel reimplantation. Although the rapidity of onset of scSSEP loss did not necessarily predict neurologic outcome, total time of scSSEP loss and time until scSSEP regeneration, as well as total aortic clamp duration, were highly significant variables predictive of neurologic deficit. This elegant study has provided the best correlation of SSEP responses and neurologic outcome available in the literature to date.

Furthermore, correlation of the prompt reversal of SSEP changes with intercostal vessel reanastomosis provides strong evidence of the worth of this maneuver in many patients if it can be accomplished in a timely fashion. In patients who had loss of SSEP with aortic clamping, neurologic outcome was much better in the subgroup in whom return of potentials could be achieved by *rapid* (i.e., less than 20 minutes) restoration of flow into the critical intercostal vessels, for example, by preservation of these vessels in a beveled proximal anastomosis of a type III aneurysm. Similar conclusions were reached by Dapunt et al. in a swine study in which localization and restoration of flow in critical intercostal vessels identified by direct scSSEP improved neurologic outcome.[18]

These studies reinforce our opinion that ischemia during the period of aortic clamping is the single most important event in the pathogenesis of cord injury and that intercostal vessel reanastomosis will generally need to be supplemented by some neuroprotective maneuver during the period of clamping to be successful.

HYPOTHERMIA FOR SPINAL CORD PROTECTION

Hypothermia is a concept that has been used throughout the evolution of cardiac and central aortic surgery. Although the neuroprotective effect of hypothermia is presumed to be secondary to decreased tissue metabolism and a generalized reduction in energy-requiring processes in the cell, the mechanism may be more complex and involve membrane stabilization and reduced release of excitatory neurotransmitters. Oxygen requirements in neural tissue are known to decrease 6% to 7% for each degree centigrade decrement in cord temperature. Hypothermia for purposes of cord protection during thoracoabdominal aneurysm surgery can be either regional, i.e., confined to the spinal cord itself, or systemic. Although profound hypothermia (15° C to 18° C) and circulatory arrest have been used successfully for many years in the correction of complex cardiac and/or aortic arch disease, enthusiasm for extending this philosophy to TAA resection has been limited, principally because of the threat of coagulopathy, pulmonary dysfunction, and massive fluid shifts.

However, Kouchoukos et al. have used this approach specifically for spinal cord protection during TAA resection.[21] They reported the use of this technique in 51 patients undergoing a variety of central aortic operations. Overall 30-day mortality was 9.8%, and spinal cord injury occurred in 6.5%. Among the 27 patients with types I, II, and III TAA, neurologic deficit occurred in 7.5% of those who survived surgery. Despite the authors' demonstration that such levels of profound hypothermia and circulatory arrest could be used for repair of TAA, the overall results, including the incidence of neurologic deficit, do not compare favorably with larger series. We believe that maintenance of nearly normal core temperature homeostasis is an important component of the overall operative management of TAA. Systemic hypothermia has been independently associated with the development of complications after elective abdominal aortic surgery.[22]

Variations of systemic hypothermia include passive moderate hypothermia where core temperature is allowed to drift to the 32° C to 34° C range by merely lowering the room temperature and allowing heat evaporation from the large surgical field. Active moderate systemic hypothermia can be achieved with the use of an in-line heat exchanger with atrial-femoral or femoral-femoral bypass. The degree of hypothermia achieved with this method is limited by the potential for cardiac arrhythmias. Two variations of regional hypothermia have been reported: direct instillation of cold perfus-

ate into the epidural or intrathecal space and intravascular cold
perfusion into isolated thoracic aortic segments with the intention
that cold perfusate will be delivered through the intercostal vessels to the spinal cord. The latter technique was originally reported
by Coles et al.[23] These investigators showed in dog experiments
that perfusion of cold Ringer's lactate into aortic segments isolated
between two clamps would rapidly diminish cord temperature to
20° C and was 100% effective in preventing paraplegia in their dog
model.

Ueno et al. showed a similar benefit of hypothermic perfusion
in a rabbit model, although no verification of the levels of hypothermia achieved in the spinal cord were reported.[24] Clinical experience with a variation of this approach was reported by Fehrenbacher et al., who used atrial-femoral bypass and passive perfusion
of isolated aortic segments in the course of sequential clamping
technique.[25] There was no verification of the degree of hypothermia achieved at the level of the spinal cord, and in the clinical setting, this method will be limited by the number and size of patent
intercostal vessels. The authors used their technique in 23 patients
with types I and II TAA and reported a 4.3% incidence of both
paraplegia and operative mortality. The principal limitations of this
method in patients relates to the previous discussion of spinal cord
blood supply. Although many animals have a "segmental" spinal
cord blood supply, i.e., multiple intercostal vessels (often those at
each segment) contribute to cord circulation, in patients few intercostals actually contribute to or become medullary arteries. Obviously, if most or all intercostals are occluded by mural thrombus,
none of the isolated aortic segment perfusate will reach the cord.
Based on our experience with the volumes of continuous perfusate required to actually cool the cord when delivered by direct epidural infusion (see later), it is difficult to conceive that any variation of the isolated aortic segment perfusion method could actually achieve meaningful cord cooling.

Experimental work with regional hypothermic perfusion delivered directly to the epidural or intrathecal space and achieving profound (less than 20° C) hypothermia has demonstrated a 100% protective effect against cord injury.[26–29] Achievement of this degree
of hypothermia, however, has generally required open laminotomy
techniques not applicable to the clinical setting. It remained for
Marsala et al. to demonstrate that a clinically applicable closed epidural infusion system that achieved moderate (26° C to 28° C) levels of cord hypothermia could be 100% effective against spinal
cord ischemia induced by double thoracic aortic clamping.[30] We

adapted this strategy and have applied it in patients since 1993. The regional hypothermia strategy is straightforward, i.e., the cord is less vulnerable to ischemic damage while its principal and/or collateral circulation is interrupted by aortic cross-clamping.

TECHNICAL CONSIDERATIONS AND CLINICAL RESULTS WITH EPIDURAL COOLING

Before specific consideration of epidural cooling, commentary relative to our overall approach to operative management of TAA is appropriate. Progress in this field is often gauged in terms of a "learning curve" in which overall results improve with accumulating experience. Such was the case at our institution when we demonstrated that operative results improved substantially after 1985 and were correlated with decreased blood turnover and decreased operative and cross-clamp times.[6] We adopted an approach along the tenets originally espoused by Crawford—stressing operative expediency and simplicity with avoidance of systemic heparin and extracorporeal bypass of any kind. Specific adjuncts to protect the kidneys (direct cold perfusion) and spinal cord (epidural cooling) and minimize visceral ischemia (recently adopted in-line mesenteric shunt)[31] complement the clamp-and-sew method. By using this approach, overall results over the past decade in 170 patients have been favorable, with operative mortality being 9% (5% in elective operations), spinal cord injury occurring in 7%, and dialysis needed in only 2.5%.[8] Thoracoabdominal aortic aneurysm distribution in this cohort has been 50% type I and II, 35% type III, and 15% type IV, and 22% had either urgent operations or frank rupture. Approximately half of those with types I, II, and III TAA treated over this interval have been managed with epidural cooling.

The mechanics of the epidural infusion system have been described previously in detail[32] and are displayed in Figure 2. The principal components of the system are a 4F epidural catheter placed at T12–L1 and advanced cephalad 4 to 5 cm, a 4F single-lumen intrathecal catheter placed at the L3–L4 level and advanced cephalad 5 cm, an infusion pump modified to permit flow rates up to 33 mL/min and connected to the epidural catheter through a coil immersed in an ice bath, and an in-line temperature sensor just proximal to the epidural catheter connection to record injectate temperature. The epidural catheter is used for both administration of local anesthetic and infusion of iced saline (4° C) perfusate. The spinal catheter permits continuous CSF temperature (CSFT) and CSF pressure (CSFP) recordings, as well as the ability to with-

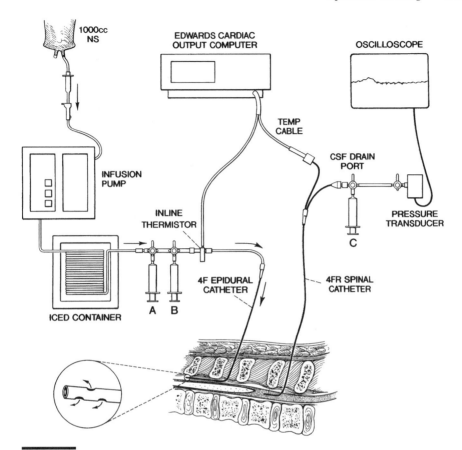

FIGURE 2.

Equipment setup for epidural cold infusion and measurement of CSF temperature and pressure. *Syringe A* is for local anesthesia, *syringe B* is for bolus doses and infusate removal, and *syringe C* is for CSF drainage. (Courtesy of Davison JK, Cambria RP, Vierra DJ, et al: Epidural cooling for regional spinal cord hypothermia during thoracoabdominal aneurysm repair. *J Vasc Surg 20:304–310, 1994.*)

draw CSF. No additional epidural drainage catheter is used because the infusate diffuses from the epidural space via nerve roots into the retroperitoneum and mediastinum.

Before the induction of general anesthesia, a sensory level is confirmed after an injection of 2% lidocaine to produce a level adequate for surgical incision. At this time, the integrity of the cooling system is confirmed with a rise in CSFP and a decrease in CSFT. Additional doses of lidocaine are given as indicated by the need for more anesthesia up until the time or aortic cross-clamping, from which time only the cold perfusate is given through the epidural. With the onset of surgery, 20 mL of CSF is removed and the epidural iced saline infusion is started at rates of 4 to 5 mL/min and adjusted to achieve a CSFT of 23° C to 25° C before aortic clamping. Selection of a target CSFT of 25° C was originally based on data from Marsala et al.[30] and correlative information with direct thermistor needles placed into the cord itself in a sheep model. In these studies we could demonstrate a gradient of cooling proceeding cephalad along the cord, but a cord substance temperature of 25° C to 28° C was achieved at the T8–L1 level when CSFT was 25° C. Core temperature in these studies was not significantly decreased, as is our experience in patients to date. Using SSEPs recorded from the upper and lower extremities, we have also demonstrated in a small number of patients that epidural cooling is associated with physiologic alterations in spinal cord function before aortic cross-clamping. With the onset on cooling, SSEPs recorded from the lower extremity are ablated as expected in the hypothermic milieu; SSEPs from the arm are maintained, thus providing further evidence of the regional distribution of the cooling effect.[33]

Intraoperative information relative to CSFT, CSFP, and core temperature in 70 patients undergoing resection of types I, II, and III TAA are displayed in Figure 3.[7] Cerebrospinal fluid pressure rises during the epidural infusion—averaging twice the baseline in our patients—and is a matter of significant concern relative to spinal cord perfusion above the level of cooling. One patient after surgery for a ruptured type I TAA manifested an atypical proximal cervicothoracic cord injury evidenced by severe bilateral arm weakness. Reliable tracings of the CSFP were lost in this patient, and we speculate that the cord injury was related to inadequate spinal cord perfusion and elevated CSFP. The thoracolumbar region of the spinal cord, which is typically vulnerable to ischemic injury, was unaffected, presumably because of the regional hypothermia.

This experience has prompted us to maintain an arbitrary 35– to 40–mm Hg gradient between the mean arterial pressure and mean CSFP by either decreasing the epidural infusion rate or increasing systemic arterial pressure. Cerebrospinal fluid drainage cannot usually be accomplished once the infusion has been started because of compression of the space. However, a characteristic pulsatile CSFP trace is seen during cooling and should be monitored for damping indicative of excessive CSFP. Epidural cooling is maintained until the distal aortic anastomosis is completed, and CSFT rapidly returns to within 1° C of core temperature by the end of the procedure. The average volume of infusate in our 70 patients was just over 1,400 mL, and the mean SCFT during aortic cross-clamping was 25° C. Other relevant intraoperative data included a visceral ischemic time that averaged 48 minutes and an aggressive posture toward reanastomosis of patient intercostal vessels in the T8–L1 region. Fifty percent of the patients had patent intercostal vessels in this zone either preserved in a beveled proximal or distal anastomosis or reconstructed with separate inclusion buttons. The anesthetic technique used permitted all patients to be evaluated in the operating room at the end of the procedure to ascertain the presence or absence of immediate neurologic deficits. The epidural catheter is used postoperatively for analgesia, and the spinal catheter is maintained for 1 to 2 days in the ICU, with CSFP maintained at less than 20 mm Hg.

Neurologic outcome in these 70 patients managed with epidural cooling was compared with that of an earlier historical control group from our institution who underwent surgery in the 3

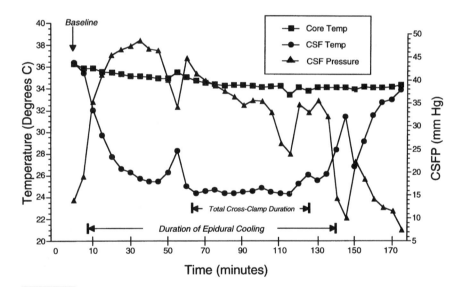

FIGURE 3.

Graphic display of mean data for CSF temperature and pressure *(CSFP)* and core temperature in 70 patients undergoing types I, II, and III thoracoabdominal aneurysm repair with the use of epidural cooling. Total cross-clamp duration refers to the interval until reperfusion of the legs. Note the mean CSF temperature of 25° C during cross-clamp and rapid return of CSF temperature to baseline after discontinuation of epidural cooling. (Courtesy of Cambria RP, Davison JK, Zannetti S, et al: Clinical experience with epidural cooling for spinal cord protection during thoracic and thoracoabdominal aneurysm repair. *J Vasc Surg* 25:234–243, 1997.)

TABLE 2.
Neurologic Deficits After Thoracoabdominal Aortic
Aneurysm Repair, 1990–1995

Patient Group	n	Observed	Predicted*	P Value
Epidural cooling	70	2 (2.9%)†	14 (20%)	0.001
Control	55	13 (23%)†	10 (17.8%)	0.48

*Predicted by using the model of Acher et al. (Acher CW, Wynn MM,
Hoch JR, et al: Combined use of cerebrospinal fluid drainage and
naloxone reduces the risk of paraplegia in thoracoabdominal aneurysm
repair. *J Vasc Surg* 19:236–246, 1994).
† $P < 0.001$ for observed deficits between the epidural group and
control.

years immediately before adoption of the epidural cooling system.
These two groups were well matched with respect to those clinical variables (aneurysm extent, acute conditions or dissection,
cross-clamp time) known to influence the risk of postoperative cord
injury. In fact, there was a higher (50% vs. 38%, $P = 0.14$) percentage of more extensive type I and II TAA in the epidural cooling group. As displayed in Table 2, there was a highly significant
reduction in the incidence of neurologic deficits in patients managed with epidural cooling when compared with historical con-
trols. Furthermore, there was a highly significant ($P = 0.001$) reduction in the incidence of neurologic deficits when compared
with that predicted with the Acher model.

It is useful to consider the entire interval (1990–1995) encompassed in our study to assess the impact of epidural cooling on
neurologic deficits after TAA repair.[7] The significant reduction in
ischemic cord complications was in large part caused by elimination of immediate total paraplegia, clearly the most devastating in
the spectrum of cord deficits. After univariate analysis of a variety
of variables tested for their association with postoperative neurologic deficit, only prolonged aortic clamp time and lack of epidural
cooling were associated with cord injury. Both these variables retained significance after the more stringent test of logistic regression analyses, with prolonged (longer than 60 minutes) visceral
clamp time having a relative risk (RR) of 4.4 (95% confidence interval [CI], 1.2 to 16.5; $P = 0.02$) and lack of epidural cooling having an RR of 9.8 (95% CI, 2 to 48; $P = 0.005$). Stated differently,
patients undergoing TAA resection at our institution during the
past 6 years were ten times more likely to sustain a postoperative

ischemic cord complication if epidural cooling was not used. This institutional experience is mirrored in the authors' recently compiled personal series of nearly 170 patients undergoing TAA repair during the past decade.

Epidural cooling has been applied (since 1993) in types I, II, and III TAA and for descending thoracic aortic resection. Nearly 100 patients with these lesions have been treated, and with the exception of the previously mentioned, probably iatrogenic cervicothoracic cord injury, only 2 deficits have occurred. Both of them occurred in delayed fashion in patients in whom technical (1 acute dissection, 1 highly calcified atheroma) considerations prevented reconstruction of the intercostals in the critical zone. One deficit was unilateral and minor with full recovery within 2 months; the other occurred on postoperative day 5 coincident with major pleural hemorrhage and shock. This patient was ambulatory with a walker in 3 months. It is unlikely that intraoperative neuroprotective adjuncts—including epidural cooling—can prevent such delayed deficits. Such observations continue to reinforce the importance of maintaining adequate arterial perfusion pressure postoperatively, especially if intercostal vessels in the critical zone have been sacrificed.

SUMMARY

The rationale for regional hypothermia relates to protection of the cord during the critical period of aortic clamping. Failure of intercostal vessel reanastomosis to have a significant impact on the complication of paraplegia may be related to the fact that revascularization simply cannot be performed rapidly enough to prevent ischemia. The data of Grabitz et al. with spinal cord evoked potential monitoring emphasized the importance of timely critical intercostal reanastomosis and suggested that the "ischemic window" for the spinal cord was less than 20 minutes.[12] Our data have led us to the conclusion that in those patients at high risk for paraplegia (i.e., resection of T8–L1 with patent intercostal vessels), some neuroprotective maneuver during the interval of aortic clamping must be added to intercostal vessel reanastomosis to prevent cord ischemic complications. The available experimental data and the clinical material reviewed herein indicate that regional cord hypothermia will fulfill this requirement.

REFERENCES

1. Svensson LG, Crawford ES, Hess KR, et al: Experience with 1509 patients undergoing thoracoabdominal aortic operations. *J Vasc Surg* 17:357–368, 1993.

2. Acher CW, Wynn MM, Hoch JR, et al: Combined use of cerebral spinal fluid drainage and naloxone reduces the risk of paraplegia in thoracoabdominal aneurysm repair. *J Vasc Surg* 19:236–246, 1994.

3. Hollier L, Money SR, Naslund TC, et al: Risk of spinal cord dysfunction in patients undergoing thoracoabdominal aortic replacement. *Am J Surg* 164:210–213, 1992.

4. Safi H, Hess KR, Randel M, et al: Cerebrospinal fluid drainage and distal aortic perfusion: Reducing neurologic complications in repair of thoracoabdominal aortic aneurysms, type I and type II. *J Vasc Surg* 23:223–228, 1996.

5. Coselli JS: Thoracoabdominal aortic aneurysms: Experience with 372 patients. *J Card Surg* 9:638–647, 1994.

6. Cambria R, Brewster DC, Moncure AC, et al: Recent experience with thoracoabdominal aneurysm repair. *Arch Surg* 124:620–624, 1989.

7. Cambria RP, Davison JK, Zannetti S, et al: Clinical experience with epidural cooling for spinal cord protection during thoracic and thoracoabdominal aneurysm repair. *J Vasc Surg* 25:234–243, 1997.

8. Cambria RP, Davison JK, Zannetti S, et al: Thoracoabdominal aneurysm repair: Perspectives over a decade with the clamp and sew technique. *Ann Surg,* in press.

9. Savader SJ, Williams GM, Trerotola SO, et al: Preoperative spinal artery localization and its relationship to postoperative neurologic complications. *Radiology* 189:165–171, 1993.

10. Kieffer E, Richard T, Chiras J, et al: Preoperative spinal cord arteriography in aneurysmal disease of the descending thoracic and thoracoabdominal aorta: Preliminary results in 45 patients. *Ann Vasc Surg* 3:34–46, 1989.

11. Svensson LG, Patel V, Robinson MF, et al: Influence of preservation or perfusion of intraoperatively identified spinal cord blood supply on motor evoked potentials and paraplegia after aortic surgery. *J Vasc Surg* 13:355–365, 1991.

12. Grabitz K, Sandmann W, Stuhmeirer K, et al: The risk of ischemic spinal cord injury in patients undergoing graft replacement for thoracoabdominal aortic aneurysms. *J Vasc Surg* 23:230–240, 1996.

13. Crawford ES, Svensson LG, Hess KR, et al: A prospective randomized study of cerebrospinal fluid drainage to prevent paraplegia after high risk surgery on the thoracoabdominal aorta. *J Vasc Surg* 13:36–46, 1991.

14. Svensson LG, Hess KR, Coselli JS, et al: Influence of segmental arteries, extent and atriofemoral bypass on postoperative paraplegia after thoracoabdominal aortic operations. *J Vasc Surg* 20:255–262, 1994.

15. Cambria RP, Giglia J: Prevention of spinal cord ischemic complications after thoracoabdominal aortic surgery. *Eur J Vasc Endovasc Surg,* in press.

16. Mauney M, Blackbourne LH, Langenburg SE, et al: Prevention of spinal cord injury after repair of the thoracic or thoracoabdominal aorta. *Ann Thorac Surg* 59:245–252, 1995.

17. Wadouh F, Arndt CF, Oppermann E, et al: The mechanism of spinal cord injury after simple and double aortic cross-clamp. *J Thorac Cardiovasc Surg 92:121–127, 1986.*

18. Dapunt O, Midulla PS, Sadeghi AM, et al: Pathogenesis of spinal cord injury during simulated aneurysm repair in a chronic animal model. *Ann Thorac Surg* 58:689–697, 1994.

19. Kazama S, Masaki Y, Maruyama S, et al: Effect of altering cerebrospinal fluid pressure on spinal cord blood flow. *Ann Thorac Surg* 38:112–115, 1994.

20. Hill A, Kalman P, Johnston KW, et al: Reversal of delayed-onset paraplegia after thoracic aortic surgery with cerebrospinal fluid drainage. *J Vasc Surg* 20:315–317, 1994.

21. Kouchoukos N, Daily BB, Rokkas CK, et al: Hypothermic bypass and circulatory arrest for operations on the descending thoracic and thoracoabdominal aorta. *Ann Thorac Surg* 60:67–77, 1995.

22. Bush HLJ, Hydo LJ, Fischer E, et al: Hypothermia during elective abdominal aortic aneurysm repair: The high risk of avoidable morbidity. *J Vasc Surg* 21:392–400, 1995.

23. Coles J, Wilson GJ, Sima AF, et al: Intraoperative management of thoracic aortic aneurysm, experimental evaluation of perfusion cooling of the spinal cord. *J Thorac Cardiovasc Surg* 85:292–299, 1983.

24. Ueno T, Furukawa K, Katayama Y, et al: Spinal cord protection: Development of a paraplegia-preventive solution. *Ann Thorac Surg* 58:116–120, 1994.

25. Fehrenbacher J, McCready RA, Hormuth DA, et al: One-stage segmental resection of extensive thoracoabdominal aneurysms with left-sided heart. *J Vasc Surg* 18:366–370, 1993.

26. Salzano R, Ellison LH, Altonji PF, et al: Regional deep hypothermia of the spinal cord protects against ischemic injury during thoracic aortic cross-clamping. *Ann Thorac Surg* 57:65–70, 1994.

27. Wisselink W, Becker MO, Nguyen JH, et al: Protecting the ischemic spinal cord during aortic clamping: The influence of selective hypothermia and spinal cord perfusion pressure. *J Vasc Surg* 19:788–795, 1994.

28. Berguer R, Porto J, Fedoronko B, et al: Selective deep hypothermia of the spinal cord prevents paraplegia after aortic cross-clamping in the dog model. *J Vasc Surg* 15:62–71, 1992.

29. Vanicky I, Marsala M, Galik J, et al: Epidural perfusion cooling protection against protracted spinal cord ischemia in rabbits. *J Neurosurg* 79:736–741, 1993.

30. Marsala M, Vanicky I, Galik J, et al: Panmyelic epidural cooling protects against ischemic spinal cord damage. *J Surg Res* 55:21–31, 1993.

31. Cambria RP, Davison JK, Giglia J: In-line mesenteric shunting reduces visceral ischemic time during thoracoabdominal aneurysm repair. *J Vasc Surg,* submitted for publication.

32. Davison JK, Cambria RP, Vierra DJ, et al: Epidural cooling for regional

spinal cord hypothermia during thoracoabdominal aneurysm repair. *J Vasc Surg* 20:304–310, 1994.

33. Lopez-Bresnahan MV, Conceicao I, Davison JK, et al: Somatosensory evoked potential changes with regional spinal cord cooling in patients undergoing thoracoabdominal aneurysm repair. *J Electroencaphalogr Clin Neurophysiol,* in press.

CHAPTER 8

Utility of Spiral CT in the Preoperative Evaluation of Patients with Abdominal Aortic Aneurysms

Mark F. Fillinger, M.D.
Assistant Professor of Surgery, Section of Vascular Surgery,
Dartmouth-Hitchcock Medical Center, Lebanon, New Hampshire

The traditional preoperative evaluation of abdominal aortic aneurysms (AAAs) includes angiography, conventional CT, or both. Angiography provides excellent images of the aortic lumen and branch vessels, but it cannot provide information about the location or thickness of an intraluminal thrombus, which makes it impossible to distinguish a normal-diameter aorta from a thrombus-filled aneurysm. Angiography is also invasive and expensive (two to three times the cost of CT). Conventional CT delineates intraluminal thrombus and the extent of the aneurysm, and can display important features such as retroaortic renal veins, inflammatory rims, retroperitoneal fibrosis, tumors, and other structures that are not depicted well by angiography. Unfortunately, conventional CT is not accurate when evaluating occlusive disease, so patients with suspected renovascular hypertension, mesenteric ischemia, or iliac occlusive disease have traditionally required angiography. When routine angiography is performed, even asymptomatic patients will have a significant number of pertinent findings.[1] Thus, in many centers, patients with AAAs often undergo angiography and CT in preoperative evaluation.

Spiral CT has dramatically changed the traditional CT evaluation. This is especially true regarding AAAs. Spiral or helical CT can acquire large quantities of data in far less time than conventional CT because data are acquired continuously while the patient moves through the scanner. Spiral CT has two major advantages:

the collimation (section thickness) can be decreased, and multiplanar reformatting into sagittal, coronal, or arbitrary planes is possible. These features are essential in the evaluation of visceral, renal, and iliac artery occlusive disease. The combination of spiral CT and multiplanar reformatting is often referred to as CT angiography, which is helpful when evaluating the extent of aortic aneurysms, the presence of visceral aneurysms, or the presence of occlusive disease.[2–6] Computed tomography angiography (CTA) is still a two-dimensional representation of a three-dimensional structure, however, and more recently three-dimensional reconstructions have been created from spiral CT data using a variety of techniques.[2, 3, 7] Initial experience suggests that three-dimensional reconstructions provide additional insight into aneurysm anatomy and a more rapid understanding of complex anatomy. We found spiral CT with three-dimensional reconstruction extremely useful in the preoperative evaluation of AAA morphology, and it has become our routine imaging method for these cases. In many respects, this imaging method appears to be more accurate than conventional methods, especially with regard to suprarenal aortic aneurysms, complex anatomy, suspected occlusive disease, and the potential for endovascular repair.

TECHNICAL CONSIDERATIONS

Although this chapter is directed at clinical applications, the technical aspects of spiral CT are key to its clinical utility, and deserve an overview. Spiral CT data acquisition occurs by rotation of the x-ray source while the gantry (table) moves in a continuous linear fashion. Advances in x-ray tube technology allow continuous x-ray beam transmission in a 360-degree arc for intervals of 30 seconds or more. Combined with linear table movement, the continuous scan path traces the classic spiral from which the technique derives its name. More importantly, this technique allows data from a large volume to be acquired rapidly—during a single breath-hold and a single contrast bolus—so motion artifacts and contrast load are greatly reduced. A typical scan might use IV contrast material injected at 2–5 mL/sec, a slice thickness (collimation) of 5 mm, a table speed of 5 mm/sec, 30–50 seconds continuous scan time, and an x-ray source that rotates 360 degrees in 1 second. The contrast level is manually or automatically monitored so the scan sequence begins at the appropriate time and location. These settings would produce a spiral CT that acquires raw data over a linear distance of 15–25 cm during a single breath-hold. These settings purposely produce overlapping sections to improve the signal-to-noise ratio without failing to scan every cubic millimeter in the volume of interest. Spiral CT is thus considered a volume imaging technique.

While spiral CT hardware is impressive, the image quality is equally dependent on software. During data acquisition, sophisticated computer algorithms allow the raw data to be stored with an x, y, and z dimension, which permits reformatting of the data into extremely thin axial sections, coronal sections, and sagittal sections. This technique is commonly referred to as multiplanar reconstructions or multiplanar reformats (MPRs, Fig 1). Maximum intensity projections (MIPs) can be constructed by choosing a viewpoint and displaying a two-dimensional projection of the maximum pixel intensity along the "line of sight," resulting in a view very similar to that of an angiogram. Three-dimensional reconstructions are also possible with the most recent spiral CT workstations. Most importantly, viewing the data from many different perspectives is possible without exposing the patient to any additional radiation or contrast material.

With regard to three-dimensional reconstructions, most CT workstations use automated computer algorithms that rely on the dramatic difference in density between the contrast-material–filled vessel lumen and surrounding structures such as thrombus. Thus, a three-dimensional image of the contrast-enhanced lumen is generated relatively quickly and easily. These automated algorithms cannot generate three-dimensional images that include thrombus or noncalcified plaque, however, because the computer cannot distinguish these anatomical features of the AAA from adjacent psoas muscle or vena cava. Calcified plaque is often erroneously included in automated three-dimensional reconstructions of the blood-flow because the algorithms cannot delineate calcified plaque from contrast-enhanced blood. Thus, the automated three-dimensional images currently generated by most spiral CT scanners are useful for evaluating tortuous vessels and AAAs with little thrombus, but they should not be used to precisely determine the extent of the aneurysm or occlusive disease in areas that contain calcified plaque.

More sophisticated three-dimensional reconstruction techniques are becoming available, however. We participated in the development of a three-dimensional imaging system capable of displaying thrombus and calcified plaque as separate objects. This involves a semi-automated process in which a skilled technician directs the computer in edge detection of structures that are less distinct or ambiguous. The process is more time- and labor-intensive, but it provides data and images that cannot be obtained

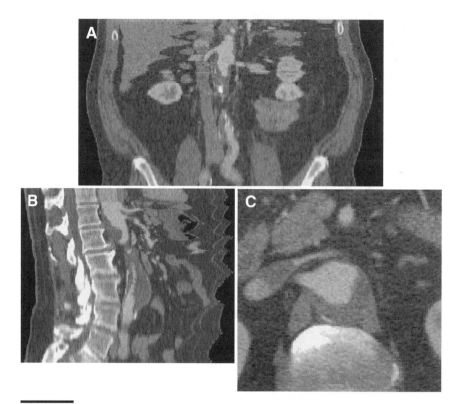

FIGURE 1.

Examples of multiplanar reconstruction or reformatting made possible by spiral CT technology. **A,** coronal reconstruction demonstrating a cross-section through the origin of the right renal artery. The left common iliac artery is also seen in this section, but much of the tortuous AAA is out of the plane shown here. Note the smooth contours at the skin edge. **B,** sagittal reformat through the celiac artery origin. The origin of the superior mesenteric artery (SMA) is also seen, but the entire SMA is seen better in another section, demonstrating the need to examine serial MPRs to obtain accurate anatomical data. Motion at the skin edge is due to the patient's inability to perform a 30-second breath-hold, thus he was allowed to take shallow breaths during the scan. Despite this, there is almost no motion in relatively fixed structures such as the aorta and spine. **C,** conventional axial CT section at the origin of the right renal artery. Note the aortic diameter compared to the diameter of the contrast-filled lumen. Examination of the coronal and axial sections makes it clear that there is no stenosis at the origin of this right renal artery.

with simpler methods. Our group and other groups working on similar three-dimensional modeling techniques (capable of displaying thrombus as a distinct structure) find this method of display extremely useful in portraying the extent of aneurysmal and occlusive disease.[3, 7]

Scrolling or "paging" through multiple axial, coronal, or sagittal cross-sections will also help clarify the anatomy. Although only limited hard copies of selected views are generally provided to surgeons, spiral CT with thin axial reconstructions over a large volume will generate hundreds of sections. Most spiral CT workstations will allow scrolling through every section in the entire dataset. Arrangements can usually be made with the radiology department so that the operating surgeon can take advantage of this capability. Usually this requires viewing the data on the day the scan is performed, in collaboration with a radiologist. Most radiology departments only archive selected hard copies, so special workstation capabilities such as scrolling through the dataset and generating MPRs or three-dimensional reconstructions are only available on the day of the scan. Even if the entire CT dataset is archived, it is time-consuming to bring the data back "on-line" for viewing on a workstation. We developed a protocol to place the entire spiral CT dataset onto a CD-ROM disk. The entire spiral CT dataset, multiplanar reformats, and an interactive three-dimensional model of the data can be viewed on a personal computer using specialized software. Unlimited access to the entire dataset is quite useful for the initial planning of AAA repair, and for detailed review immediately prior to or during the procedure.

Hopefully this brief discussion of spiral CT technology will make it easier to understand how the images presented in this chapter are made possible. Discussion of more technical issues such as "pitch" (ratio of table speed to slice thickness), interpolation algorithms, acquisition protocols, and reconstruction algorithms are beyond the scope of this text. Several excellent texts and articles are available for the interested reader. The remainder of this chapter will be devoted to the clinical utility of the unique images made possible by spiral CT technology.

CLINICAL CONSIDERATIONS

There are a number of anatomic features that are crucial to the appropriate planning of AAA repair: the precise proximal and distal extent of the aneurysm (especially the presence of juxtarenal or suprarenal extension); occlusive or aneurysmal disease in the visceral, renal, or iliac arteries; multiple renal arteries or accessory renal arteries; duplicate or left-sided vena cava; vascular anomalies including horseshoe kidney; and aortic dissections. Many of these anatomical features can be dealt with at repair, but it is safer and more efficient if the surgeon knows about them prior to the procedure. Many of these structures can alter the operative plan or the risk-benefit ratio of the procedure. Features such as retroaortic renal veins, patency of the inferior mesenteric artery (IMA), the number and location of patent lumbar arteries, and the degree of calcified or noncalcified plaque at the sites of anastomoses can also be important when planning an AAA repair. Traditionally, delineation of all the aforementioned anatomical features required a combination of conventional CT and angiography, but state-of-the-art spiral CT and/or three-dimensional reconstruction may now be all that is necessary in most cases.

EXTENT OF THE ANEURYSM

Perhaps the single most important morphologic consideration for repair of an aortic aneurysm is the proximal and distal extent of disease. In Figure 1, C, it is apparent that the aorta is still aneurysmal at the level of the right renal artery. It is also apparent from Figure 1, C that an angiogram of the contrast-filled lumen would not reveal the aneurysmal nature of the aorta at this level, because much of the aneurysm is occupied by thrombus. Thus, CT is generally recognized as the best imaging modality for ascertaining the proximal and distal extent of an aortic aneurysm. Spiral CT offers distinct advantages over conventional CT in this respect, however, because the data may be viewed from different perspectives via MPRs and three-dimensional reconstructions. Three-dimensional reconstructions can be especially helpful in determining the extent of aneurysmal disease and the locations for optimal cross-clamp placement.[2, 3] In Figure 2, it is immediately obvious that the patient has separate thoracic and abdominal aortic aneurysms, and that repair of the thoracic aneurysm will require a clamp placed just above the level of the celiac artery (which is precisely what was found at surgery). This demonstrates how a three-dimensional reconstruction can facilitate recognition of aneurysm morphology and extent, especially when the reconstructions include thrombus and not just the contrast-enhanced vessel lumen.

In a recent series from our center, 55 patients with AAA underwent spiral CT, including MPRs and three-dimensional reconstruction. In this group, there were 14 patients with aneurysmal involvement of the suprarenal aorta. Three-dimensional reconstructions were created and assessed without access to radiology reports from the initial spiral CT scan. Other imaging studies (duplex, angiography) were assessed with access to spiral CT findings, but not three-dimensional reconstructions. In this subset of patients with suprarenal aneurysms, conventional CT and angiography failed to predict the true extent of the aneurysm and the opti-

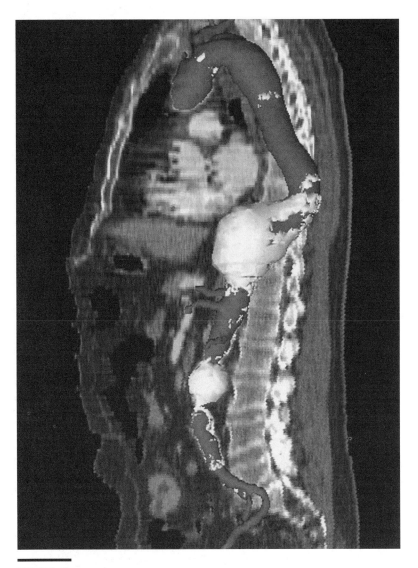

FIGURE 2.

Patient with separate thoracic and abdominal aortic aneurysms. Here a sagittal section has been "dropped into" a three-dimensional model to add context. Thrombus and calcified plaque are displayed in lighter shades of grey on the model. Note the location where the SMA ends on the model but continues in the sagittal section. Note also that the three-dimensional model immediately conveys information that would require a large number of axial, sagittal, and coronal sections (although a significant amount of information is lost in this black-and-white reproduction of a color three-dimensional model). For more detailed information, it is best to view magnified views of the multiplanar reformats or magnified and rotated views of the three-dimensional model with and without thrombus or plaque.

mal cross-clamp location in the majority of cases. In each case, however, preoperative spiral CT with three-dimensional reconstruction revealed the correct proximal and distal extent of the aneurysm when compared to operative findings.[7] Spiral CT with three-dimensional reconstruction was also superior to spiral CT alone. It has been suggested that CT overestimates the extent of aneurysmal disease, but thus far, we have not predicted a suprarenal aneurysm when an infrarenal AAA was present.

Although determining the extent of the aneurysm is extremely important with conventional AAA repair, the operation can usually be modified to account for unexpected extension of an aneurysm proximally or distally. In endovascular AAA repair, however, corrections during graft delivery are not possible, and the graft length and diameter must be determined prior to graft deployment. More importantly, endovascular AAA repair is guided by angiography instead of direct vision, making preoperative determination of the extent of disease even more important. Three-dimensional reconstructions can be extremely helpful in this respect, especially when the thrombus is included in the reconstruction. Figure 3 demonstrates how angiography and three-dimensional reconstruction of only the contrast-enhanced lumen generally underestimate the extent of the aneurysm, which would be a critical error when planning an endovascular AAA repair. Multiplanar reformats and three-dimensional reconstruction of spiral CT data can also be used to perform preoperative diameter and length measurements for endovascular grafts,[8] but this is beyond the scope of this text.

Another important aspect of preoperative evaluation for AAAs is the evaluation of aneurysmal disease in the iliac arteries, either as an extension of the AAA or as isolated disease. In many cases, conventional CT has been poor in this regard, and even relatively recent series have reported error rates of 16% for depicting iliac aneurysms.[9] However, groups using spiral CT with MPRs alone have noted accuracy of over 90% for the depiction of iliac aneurysms.[5] In our series of over 50 AAAs evaluated with spiral CT including MPRs and three-dimensional reconstruction, we have not missed a single iliac aneurysm as evaluated during open repair.

OCCLUSIVE DISEASE OF THE AORTIC BRANCHES

Another key aspect in the preoperative evaluation of AAAs is the extent of occlusive disease in aortic branch vessels. Patients with suspected iliac, renal, or visceral occlusive disease have always required angiography prior to AAA repair, because evaluation of occlusive disease has been a traditional downfall of conventional

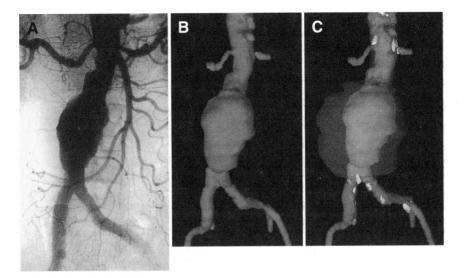

FIGURE 3.

A, anteroposterior view of an angiogram performed on a patient being evaluated for AAA repair. Note the irregularity of the aortic lumen below the renal arteries and the apparent presence of a distal cuff below the AAA. **B,** anteroposterior view of a three-dimensional reconstruction from spiral CT data portraying blood flow only. Note the similarity to the angiogram. **C,** the same three-dimensional reconstruction with solid blood flow *(grey),* solid calcified plaque *(white),* and transparent thrombus *(shaded with dots),* demonstrating that the aneurysm ends at the aortic bifurcation—there is no distal cuff of normal diameter aorta. The IMA appears to fill from the aorta on angiography, but at surgery it was found to be occluded at its origin, as noted in the three-dimensional reconstruction.

CT.[10] With conventional CT, tube overheating problems limited the number of sections that could be obtained and the volume of the body that could be covered by the scan. Therefore, fewer axial sections were obtained in the visceral and renal segments, and very few sections were obtained in the iliac segment. The paucity of sections and the tortuosity of the vessels thus made evaluation of occlusive disease difficult.

Because of the technical considerations previously mentioned, spiral CT can cover a large patient volume and still provide large numbers of thin multiplanar sections. This ability is key to the evaluation of occlusive disease. Large numbers of thin axial sections make it more likely that a stenosis will be clearly seen on axial sections alone, and this technique also improves the quality of multiplanar reformats and three-dimensional reconstructions. Thus, with appropriate scan protocols and adequate timing of the contrast load, evaluation of iliac occlusive disease with spiral CT is far superior to conventional CT and rivals angiography.[5] In many cases, identification of occlusive disease does not even require multiple views (Fig 4, A–C). In preliminary comparisons at our institution, angiography accurately depicted iliac artery occlusive

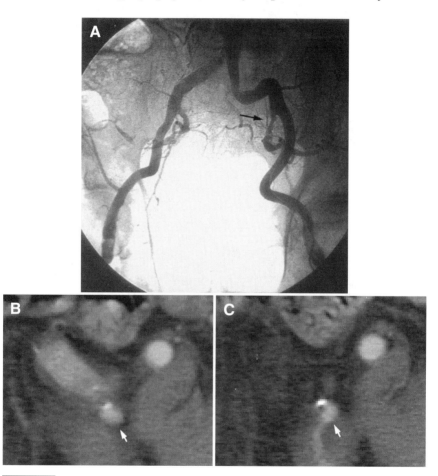

FIGURE 4.

A, angiogram demonstrating left internal iliac artery occlusive disease *(arrow).* **B,** proximal left internal iliac artery *(arrow)* on axial CT is relatively free of occlusive disease. **C,** axial CT section distal to the section in Figure 4, B demonstrates thick plaque encroaching the lumen of the left internal iliac artery *(arrow),* which corresponds to the stenosis seen on angiography. In this particular patient, axial sections alone are sufficient to demonstrate occlusive disease in the left internal iliac artery. Multiplanar reformats and three-dimensional reconstruction could further elucidate the occlusive disease and potentially eliminate the need for angiography in this patient.

disease with 50% or greater stenosis in 22 of 28 cases (79%), spiral CT with axial sections alone was accurate in 22 of 28 cases (79%), and spiral CT with MPRs and three-dimensional reconstruction was correct in all 28 cases.

The evaluation of occlusive disease in the renal and mesenteric vessels, however, is more difficult than evaluation of iliac occlusive disease. The vessels are smaller, the stenotic areas are often quite short, and the vessels may be oriented at odd angles relative to conventional axial sections. Again, spiral CT is superior to conventional CT because of the availability of extremely thin (1–2 mm) axial sections and multiplanar reconstructions. We generally use a protocol that consists of 3-mm collimation, with 1-mm axial reconstructions (reformats) through the visceral segment. These vessels are best evaluated by views or sections perpendicular to the long axis of the vessel. Thus, the renal arteries are best evaluated with axial, coronal, and three-dimensional reconstructions, while the celiac and superior mesenteric arteries are best depicted in axial, sagittal, and three-dimensional reconstructions. Computed tomography artifacts are possible, including motion artifacts (patient movement during the scan) and partial volume averaging artifact (e.g., signal averaging from dense structures such as calcium causing a small rim of adjacent thrombus to have the appearance of contrast-enhanced blood flow). Multiplanar reconstructions are often helpful in this regard, however, and we are much more confident when a stenosis appears consistently in multiple views. Figure 5, A–D demonstrates the utility of spiral CT with three-dimensional reconstruction for the evaluation of renal artery stenosis. We have found these techniques to be quite accurate in a pilot study correlating angiography with spiral CT and three-dimensional reconstruction. Evaluating the renal and visceral arteries for stenoses greater than 50%, spiral CT with MPRs and interactive three-dimensional reconstructions had an accuracy of 97% relative to operative findings, which compared well with the 93% accuracy of angiography. Other investigators have also found a high degree of accuracy for renal artery stenoses using spiral CT and MPRs alone,[4, 5, 11, 12] although sensitivities in the 90% range are not universal.[6, 13] In general, however, the accuracy of spiral CT is uniformly superior to reported values for conventional CT.[10] Depiction of visceral artery stenosis appears to be very accurate in most studies.[5, 6] Clearly, one should not rely solely on three-dimensional reconstructions for assessment of renal or visceral artery stenoses.[13] It should be emphasized that in our experience, a complete evaluation of visceral or renal artery occlusive disease should include a thorough study of all available axial, coronal, and

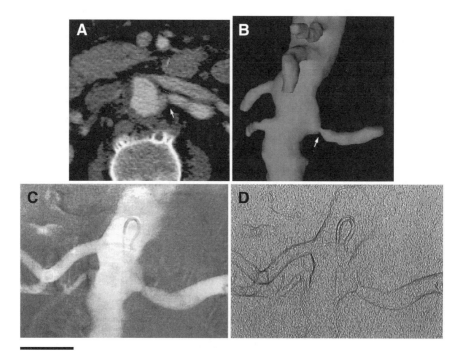

FIGURE 5.

Left renal artery stenosis demonstrated by several different imaging modalities: **A,** axial cross-section from a spiral CT shows stenosis *(arrow)*. **B,** three-dimensional reconstruction from the spiral CT data shows stenosis *(arrow)*. **C,** digital subtraction angiogram. **D,** digital subtraction angiogram using an edge enhancement technique. Note the right lower pole accessory renal artery, which is depicted in all four views (the axial CT section demonstrates only the lower portion; the origin of the accessory renal is demonstrated in a more proximal section).

sagittal sections, including magnified views. If three-dimensional reconstructions are available, magnified and rotated views with and without plaque are helpful. Appropriate scanning protocols and detailed evaluation are needed to obtain high-quality results. If this latest generation technology continues to produce excellent results, however, angiography will rarely be necessary for preoperative evaluation of AAAs.

ACCESSORY RENAL ARTERIES AND INFERIOR MESENTERIC ARTERY PATENCY

Another area that has traditionally been difficult for conventional CT is the evaluation of accessory renal arteries and the inferior mesenteric artery (IMA). Because of the advantages previously outlined, spiral CT is quite good at depicting the presence of these vessels and determining whether they are patent or not. Three-dimensional reconstruction is also helpful in this regard, but the key to accuracy in imaging these vessels involves very thin axial reconstructions and a person who is willing to scroll through every single axial section looking for the presence of these small vessels. With 1–2 mm reconstructions, a typical spiral CT scan for AAA evaluation will generate hundreds of axial sections. It is not adequate to review the 20 to 40 hard copies that might be printed out from a single scan. It is necessary for the radiologist or surgeon to sit down at the CT workstation and review every single axial section. In our institution, the surgeon uses special software to review each individual section on a personal computer (see Technical Considerations). Automated three-dimensional reconstruction algorithms are unreliable in this situation because the contrast may be poor in these small vessels (another form of partial volume averaging).

Our current scan protocol uses 3-mm collimation through the visceral/renal segment, 1-mm axial reconstructions, scrolling through each of the axial sections (including magnified views when necessary), use of multiplanar reformatting to view the vessels in two or three planes, and three-dimensional reconstructions capable of displaying the blood flow, thrombus, and calcified plaque as separate objects. The separate objects in our three-dimensional models also can be viewed individually, and rotated to view the structure from any angle. This technique has excellent accuracy in depicting the number, location, and patency of accessory renal arteries. When compared to operative findings in over 50 cases, we identified all patent accessory renal arteries (although the illustration was not chosen for this aspect, an accessory renal artery can be noted in Figure 5). Other groups have noted accuracies of 96% to 100% in the demonstration of accessory renal arteries.[4, 13, 14] We found this technique to be far more accurate than angiography in the determination of IMA patency, with only one error in over 50 cases. Inferior mesenteric artery patency is demonstrated in Figure 3 where the IMA appears to originate from the aorta on angiography but not on the three-dimensional reconstruction. In this case, the IMA was indeed occluded at its origin in the aortic lumen, and filled via collateral vessels.

ASSOCIATED STRUCTURES

Computed tomography traditionally helps in the detection of unusual structures such as horseshoe kidneys, retroaortic renal vein, circumaortic renal vein, and duplicate or left-sided vena cava[9]; because of technical advantages, spiral CT is excellent for detection of these anomalies. Figure 6 demonstrates how a spiral CT section

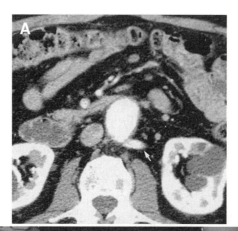

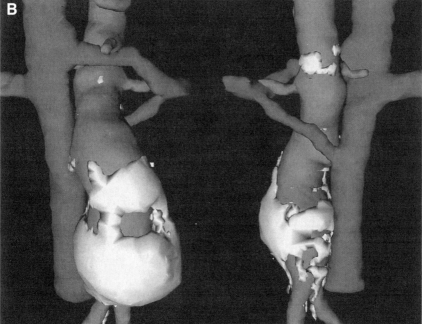

FIGURE 6.

A, axial cross-section demonstrating an apparent retroaortic renal vein *(arrow).*
B, three-dimensional reconstruction demonstrating the course and location of this
circumaortic renal vein from anterior and posterior views. Contrast-enhanced arterial blood flow and venous blood flow are both portrayed in dark grey, while
thrombus and calcified plaque are in lighter grey (in this black-and-white reproduction of a color model). The circumaortic nature of this vein could be determined by scrolling rapidly through multiple thin axial sections, but the location
and course of the vein are understood much more rapidly and easily on the three-
dimensional reconstruction.

depicts an apparent retroaortic renal vein, and how three-dimensional reconstruction can make this structure much more obvious in relation to its size and course around the aortic neck. Although these structures can be dealt with at surgery, it is certainly advantageous to know about them preoperatively. In the case of left-sided vena cava or duplicate vena cava, knowledge of the structure may change the approach from retroperitoneal to transperitoneal. Thus, spiral CT is extremely helpful in identifying these structures, and the addition of three-dimensional reconstruction can further aid planning. We found that spiral CT with MPRs and interactive three-dimensional reconstructions can accurately identify the number and location of patent lumbar arteries, and the degree of calcified or noncalcified plaque at the sites of anastomoses. Although these features will be discovered at surgery, they can be important when planning an AAA repair. This is especially true for repair of thoracoabdominal aneurysms or other complex procedures.

SUMMARY

In early clinical use, we have found spiral CT to be extremely useful for the preoperative evaluation of AAA morphology. Techniques such as multiplanar reformatting and three-dimensional reconstruction are helpful in many cases and crucial in others. There are a number of anatomical features that range from critically important to extremely helpful when planning an AAA repair: the precise proximal and distal extent of the aneurysm (especially the presence of juxtarenal or suprarenal extension); occlusive or aneurysmal disease in the visceral, renal, or iliac arteries; multiple renal arteries or accessory renal arteries; duplicate or left-sided vena cava; retroaortic renal veins, and patency of the IMA. Many of these anatomical features can be dealt with at surgery, but it is safer and more efficient if the surgeon knows about them prior to the procedure. Many of these structures can alter the operative plan or the risk-benefit ratio of the procedure. Traditionally, delineation of all the aforementioned anatomical features required a combination of conventional CT and angiography, but state-of-the-art spiral CT with MPRs may be all that is necessary in many cases. The addition of three-dimensional reconstruction can provide further information, especially if thrombus and calcified plaque are depicted as separate objects. Access to a CT workstation or specialized software will be helpful for most anatomical features, and crucial for evaluating visceral occlusive disease, accessory renal arteries, and IMAs. With appropriate protocols, spiral CT is superior to angiography in the evaluation of patients with suprarenal aortic aneurysms. We believe this imaging method is also superior when evaluating the potential for endovascular repair, for delineating complex anatomy, and for the initial evaluation of suspected occlusive disease. As this technology becomes more widely available and more thoroughly evaluated, it is likely to replace angiography in the routine preoperative evaluation of patients with abdominal aortic aneurysms. Angiography will be reserved for highly selected patients and become oriented toward a therapeutic rather than a diagnostic role.

ACKNOWLEDGMENT

We acknowledge Medical Media Systems, West Lebanon, New Hampshire (including Peter J. Robbie, MFA, S D. Pieper, Ph.D., Michael A. McKenna, Ph.D., David T. Chen, Ph.D., and Robyn E. Mosher, MSE), for providing grant/research support, novel software, and technical assistance, which enabled construction of the three-dimensional images displayed here. We also thank Robert F. Jeffery, M.D. (Department of Radiology) who has diligently worked on optimizing spiral CT protocols for our institution and provided technical assistance in downloading spiral CT data for three-dimensional reconstructions.

REFERENCES

1. Brewster DC, Retana A, Waltman AC, et al: Angiography in the management of aneurysms of the abdominal aorta. Its value and safety. *N Engl J Med* 292:822–825, 1975.
2. Rubin GD, Walker PJ, Dake MD, et al: Three-dimensional spiral computed tomographic angiography: An alternative imaging modality for the abdominal aorta and its branches. *J Vasc Surg* 18:656–665, 1993.
3. Balm R, Eikelboom BC, van Leeuwen MS, et al: Spiral CT-angiography of the aorta. *Eur J Vasc Surg* 8:544–551, 1994.
4. Van Hoe L, Baert AL, Gryspeerdt S, et al: Supra- and juxtarenal aneurysms of the abdominal aorta: Preoperative assessment with thin-section spiral CT. *Radiology* 198:443–448, 1996.
5. Raptopoulos V, Rosen MP, Kent KC, et al: Sequential helical CT angiography of aortoiliac disease. *AJR* 166:1347–1354, 1996.
6. Cikrit DF, Harris VJ, Hemmer CG, et al: Comparison of spiral CT scan and arteriography for evaluation of renal and visceral arteries. *Ann Vasc Surg* 10:109–116, 1996.
7. Fillinger MF, McKenna MA, Walsh DB, et al: Utility of spiral CT with three-dimensional reconstruction in the evaluation and management of suprarenal aortic aneurysms, submitted for publication.
8. Fillinger MF, Robbie PJ, McKenna MA, et al: The "virtual" graft: Pre-

Moving?

I'd like to receive my *Advances in Vascular Surgery* without interruption.
Please note the following change of address, effective:

Name: _____

New Address: _____

_____

City: _____ State: _____ Zip: _____

Old Address: _____

_____

City: _____ State: _____ Zip: _____

Reservation Card

Yes, I would like my own copy of *Advances in Vascular Surgery.* Please begin my subscription with the current edition according to the terms described below.* I understand that I will have 30 days to examine each annual edition. If satisfied, I will pay just $77.95 plus sales tax, postage and handling (price subject to change without notice).

Name: _____

Address: _____

City: _____ State: _____ Zip: _____

Method of Payment
○ Visa   ○ Mastercard   ○ AmEx   ○ Bill me   ○ Check (in US dollars, payable to Mosby, Inc.)

Card number: _____ Exp date: _____

Signature: _____

LS-0908

*Your *Advances* Service Guarantee:

When you subscribe to *Advances*, we'll send you an advance notice of future volumes about two months before they publish. This automatic notice system is designed to take up as little of your time as possible. If you do not want *Advances*, the advance notice makes it quick and easy for you to let us know your decision, and you will always have at least 20 days to decide. If we don't hear from you, we'll send you the new volume as soon as it's available. And, of course, *Advances* is yours to examine free of charge for 30 days (postage, handling and applicable sales tax are added to each shipment.).

BUSINESS REPLY MAIL
FIRST CLASS MAIL   PERMIT No. 762   CHICAGO, IL

POSTAGE WILL BE PAID BY ADDRESSEE

Chris Hughes
Mosby-Year Book, Inc.
161 N. Clark Street
Suite 1900
Chicago, IL 60601-9981

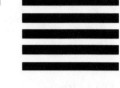

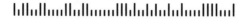

BUSINESS REPLY MAIL
FIRST CLASS MAIL   PERMIT No. 762   CHICAGO, IL

POSTAGE WILL BE PAID BY ADDRESSEE

Chris Hughes
Mosby-Year Book, Inc.
161 N. Clark Street
Suite 1900
Chicago, IL 60601-9981

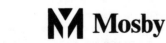

Dedicated to publishing excellence

operative simulation of endovascular grafts using spiral CT with interactive three-dimensional reconstructions. *J Endovasc Surg* 4:10, 1997.

9. Todd GJ, Nowygrod R, Benvenisty A, et al: The accuracy of CT scanning in the diagnosis of abdominal and thoracoabdominal aortic aneurysms. *J Vasc Surg* 13:302–310, 1991.

10. Salaman RA, Shandall A, Morgan RH, et al: Intravenous digital subtraction angiography versus computed tomography in the assessment of abdominal aortic aneurysm. *Br J Surg* 81:661–663, 1994.

11. Galanski M, Prokop M, Chavan A, et al: Renal arterial stenoses: Spiral CT angiography. *Radiology* 189:185–192, 1993.

12. Kaatee R, Beek FJ, Verschuyl EJ, et al: Atherosclerotic renal artery stenosis: Ostial or truncal? *Radiology* 199:637–640, 1996.

13. Rubin GD, Dake MD, Napel S, et al: Spiral CT of renal artery stenosis: Comparison of three-dimensional rendering techniques. *Radiology* 190:181–189, 1994.

14. Costello P, Gaa J: Spiral CT angiography of abdominal aortic aneurysms. *Radiographics* 15:397–406, 1995.

CHAPTER 9

Laparoscopic Aortic Surgery

Carlos R. Gracia, M.D., F.A.C.S.

Director, California Laparoscopic Institute, San Ramon Regional Medical Center, San Ramon, California

Yves-Marie Dion, M.D., M.Sc., F.A.C.S., F.R.C.S.C.

Associate Professor of Surgery, Centre Hospitalier Universitaire de Québec, Pavillon St-François d'Assise, Université Laval, Québec, Québec, Canada

During the past 50 years, a wide range of options for therapeutic management of aortoiliac disease has evolved. Such methods include anatomical (direct reconstructive procedures on the aortoiliac vessels), extraanatomic (indirect bypass grafts that avoid normal anatomical pathways), or nonoperative catheter-based endoluminal approaches to treatment of occlusive lesions by a remote, minimally invasive access to the arterial system.[1]

Currently, confusion exists due to differences in reported early and late results associated with the various therapeutic modalities. No single option for inflow revascularization is ideal or applicable to all cases. However, for most patients with diffuse aortoiliac occlusive disease, aortobifemoral (ABF) grafts remain the most durable and functionally effective means of revascularization and should continue to be rightfully regarded as the basis of comparison with other options.[1]

Over the past few years, minimally invasive surgical (MIS) approaches using laparoscopy have revolutionized the practice of surgery. The proclaimed advantages of laparoscopic surgery, such as diminished postoperative pain, decreased hospital stay, and earlier return to work have been documented.[2–5] Laparoscopic surgery is beneficial in a growing number of surgical procedures, many of which have centered around gastrointestinal, gynecologic, urologic, and general thoracic procedures. One of the newest applications of laparoscopic surgery has been in the field of vascular surgery.

Currently, minimally invasive vascular techniques are primarily endoluminal and include angioplasty, stent placement, and angioscopy, yet vascular surgeons have been slow in adopting MIS laparoscopy. This is due largely to the technical challenges imparted by the fundamentals of vascular surgery: 1) exposure, 2) vascular control, 3) vascular occlusion, 4) anastomosis of vessels and/or grafts, and 5) hemostasis. It is a difficult and stressful process to meet these challenges in the remote, hands-off operating system inherent in laparoscopy. Minimally invasive surgical technology advancements for laparoscopic application to vascular reconstruction have lagged significantly behind those that have helped its application in gastrointestinal laparoscopy.

Although in their infancy, laparoscopic vascular procedures have been performed on patients. We will review the early experimental and developmental aspects of this approach and its current successful application in clinical settings.

AORTOILIAC OCCLUSIVE DISEASE

EARLY EXPERIENCES

From 1991 through 1992, some of the earliest work on the application of evolving laparoscopic knowledge and skills to vascular surgery was carried out in Quebec, Canada by Dion, et al. Laboratory work to evaluate possible access and exposure of the aorta utilized an original abdominal wall lifting device (Laborie Surgical, Ltd) in the porcine model. Considerable concerns were raised regarding the ability to apply suction under conditions of pneumoperitoneum. There were additional concerns regarding venous air embolism while working near the major venous structures in the retroperitoneum under insufflation. A gasless approach not only eliminated these concerns, but also obviated early instrumentation problems with occlusive clamps and needle drivers, which had to be inserted in this model through blunt ports without concern for leakage of pneumoperitoneum.

This early experimental work led to the conclusion that exposure and surgery of the aorta via laparoscopy was feasible. Early instrument design ensued with standard vascular instrumentation adapted for laparoscopic application. The final result of this developmental work was the first actual application of laparoscopy to major vascular reconstructive surgery consisting of an aorto-femoral bypass (AFB) graft in humans, in March of 1993, by a surgical team led by Dr. Yves Dion of Quebec.[6] This early case was followed by four more AFBs.[7] All patients demonstrated improved postoperative courses characterized by early ambulation with less pain and less need for analgesics. Operative details included the use of pneumoperitoneum with a transperitoneal approach and all of the dissection, control, insertion, and tunneling of graft was completed laparoscopically. A small mini-laparotomy was performed to construct an end-to-side proximal anastomosis. These cases were therefore more precisely "laparoscopic-assisted."

Clinical work by Behrens and Herde[8] ensued with similar utilization of a transperitoneal route. However, an abdominal wall lift was used to create and maintain the working cavity. A variety of cases were performed, including one AFB, one aortoiliac endarterectomy, and two iliofemoral bypasses. Again, a mini-laparotomy was used not only as a facilitator for vascular suturing, but also as an avenue to provide small bowel retraction. A faster postoperative recovery with less pain was observed in these patients. This experience was also laparoscopic-assisted, and as observed in Quebec, these early experiences demonstrated reproduction of the standard operative approach for the aortoiliac arteriosclerotic occlusive disease in each circumstance. They used MIS in place of the standard incision. All patients demonstrated improved and shortened postoperative courses when compared to the traditional incisional approach.[7, 8] Important issues also were being identified during these early experiences. Would a gasless or more traditional gas-insufflation technique be best? If insufflation proved best, what are the issues with respect to the risk of gas embolism? Also, these experiences were transperitoneal and they proved to be time-consuming with much of the effort involved in maintaining small-bowel retraction. Therefore, would a retroperitoneal route be better? Finally, these experiences were also laparoscopic-assisted. The reason for the mini-laparotomy was to perform a continuous sutured vascular anastomosis, a task considered tedious and difficult with current endoscopic instrumentation. Would a totally laparoscopic approach eliminate "mini" incisions and solve some of the challenges associated with this type of surgery? Clearly more laboratory work was required.

EXPERIMENTAL WORK

The limitations of the laparoscopic-assisted approach became readily apparent. With increasing thickness of the abdominal wall, the incisions must increase in size to maintain comparable exposure and any advantages sought by minimizing trauma from the access are compromised. Dion completed additional work between 1993 and 1994 to evaluate a totally laparoscopic approach, which also included the feasibility of laparoscopic vascular suturing with pneumoperitoneum. A canine model, under CO_2 insufflation, was used where a lengthy 2 cm aortotomy was performed with a side-biting Satinsky style clamp (adapted for laparoscopy). A Hemashield (Bard) vascular prosthesis was sutured into this aortotomy as a hemostatic patch with running monofilament suture performed totally laparoscopically. This confirmed that standard vascular maneuvers, such as occlusion, opening of the vessel and direct suturing could be successfully undertaken in a totally laparoscopic environment with pneumoperitoneum.

Other investigators were also looking at the challenges of applying laparoscopy to vascular surgery. In 1995, Ahn et al.[9] reported a series of animal experiments in which 13 laparoscopic dissections proceeded via a transperitoneal approach. Seven aortofemoral bypass procedures were completed with this approach and three additional procedures were completed using a retroperitoneal approach. These procedures were performed under carbon dioxide pneumoperitoneum. Anastomoses were completed in end-to-side fashion using a combination of interrupted laparoscopic sutures and clips in five animals, with the other five being completed in end-to-end fashion with a custom-made non-sutured graft.

Another experience was reported by Jones et al.[10] in 1996 whereby transperitoneal and retroperitoneal approaches were both evaluated. In the transperitoneal approach, a mini-laparotomy was used along with an abdominal wall lift, while in the retroperitoneal approach serial balloon dissection opened the retroperitoneum while the abdominal wall lift device again maintained the working space. Overall, ten aortofemoral procedures were performed with five animals used for each different approach. The anastomoses were performed via the mini-laparotomy and the overall experience demonstrated acceptable clamp and overall operative times. The laparoscopic technique-related complications in this experience pertained to creation of the pneumoperitoneum and retraction of small bowel and occurred only in the group that underwent the transperitoneal approach. These investigators reported that both approaches were effective for gasless laparoscopic-assisted exposure of the aorta. However, they noted that the retroperitoneal approach facilitated bowel retraction by using the intact peritoneal sac.

Three important concepts began to unfold. First, a gasless approach seemed promising for the previously outlined reasons, yet the three-dimensional compressing effect of gas insufflation proved potentially desirable. The safety of its use requires further investigation. Where gasless technique would represent an alternative to pneumoperitoneum when surgery is performed in localized regions of the abdomen, such as in the pelvis or upper abdomen, its application to the peritoneal cavity at large can be a problem. During gasless surgery, the compressing effect of carbon dioxide under normal working pressures (12–15 mmHg) is not present and the small bowel tends to occupy more space in the abdominal cavity. Variation in patients' body size and morphology could make working under a gasless environment more difficult.

Second, laparoscopic-assisted by mini-laparotomy ultimately may prove very limiting. It is difficult to make small incisions in patients with thick or obese abdominal walls. With increasing thickness of abdominal walls, the incisions must increase in length to maintain exposure, proportionately reducing advantages inherent in minimizing trauma from access. As a result, we thought that a completely laparoscopic approach ultimately may be more reproducible and overcome limitations imposed by small incisions. This approach obviously requires resolution of major technical challenges, along with development of appropriate instrumentation for these tasks.

Finally, the third issue centered on the optimal approach, transperitoneal vs. retroperitoneal. The early human clinical experience of Dion et al. confirmed the difficulty of the transperitoneal route with respect to bowel retraction in that aortic dissection and end-to-side aortoprosthetic anastomosis proved quite tedious. The solution may lie in a retroperitoneal approach since the peritoneal sac could function as an organ retractor and provide excellent major vessel exposure.

The first reported work toward the consistent use of a retroperitoneal approach was the animal series reported by Dion et al.[11] in 1995. While the anterior approach of Schumacker[12] was initially used, it was abandoned for a lateral approach to access the retroperitoneum. With the piglets in the right lateral decubitus position, retroperitoneal dissection (aided by balloon dissectors) allowed creation of a retroperitoneal space. The aorta was visualized and dissected from the left renal artery distally. Abdominal wall suspension (Laparolift, Origin Medsystems) was then used due to concerns regarding the use of suction and the lack of complete instrumentation to work in a sealed gas environment. Totally laparoscopic aortoprosthetic anastomoses were performed. However, the exposure of the femoral vessels and tunneling of the prosthetic graft to the groins required that the animal be turned to a more supine position to complete the aortobifemoral bypass procedure.

Despite the success of the previous experience, it was apparent that translation of this model to actual human application would require the undesirable task of having to turn the patient from a lateral position, which would preclude access for proximal control. Also, it could allow for breaks in the sterile technique. It is important to consider the consequences of aortic prosthetic infection and bleeding to avoid these risks. Could their approach be modified to allow the patient to remain in a supine rather than lateral position? This would provide access for proximal control or maneuvering if necessary, and for exposure of the femoral arteries without concern for the potential risks involved in turning the patient.

An anterolateral laparoscopic approach with the subject supine (Fig 1) was subsequently performed and reported by Dion and Gracia.[13] The goal was not only to reproduce the exposure and control obtained with the lateral approach, but also to completely expose and control the distal aorta and iliac arteries. Exposure and control of the inferior mesenteric and lumbar arteries was also necessary to prevent significant bleeding, which could rapidly obscure the operative laparoscopic view.

Despite the issues raised previously, an abdominal wall lift was used in both these retroperitoneal experiences.[11, 13] At the time, the abdominal wall lifting device maintained the working cavity in case of prolonged suctioning or port leakage. It also allowed insertion of more conventional instrumentation or multiple tools at a port site since a gas seal was no longer necessary and gas-sealed instruments were not available. However, the retroperitoneal approach was resolving the difficulties encountered by the previous transperitoneal experience, both experimental and clinical, in that bowel retraction was simplified. These procedures were now being completed safely, without the aid of mini-laparotomy for any portion of the procedure, including construction of end-to-end aortoprosthetic anastomosis with running monofilament suture.

In the technique developed by Dion and Gracia,[13] the aorta was approached in different fashions to reproduce occlusive disease as well as aneurysmal disease. In the former, after proximal occlusion and oversewing of the distal aorta, the aorta was transected and an end-to-end aortoprosthetic anastomosis was performed. In the latter, an aneurysmal model was used wherein proximal and distal control was established, and the aorta was opened longitudinally. The lumbar arteries were controlled external to the aorta and over-

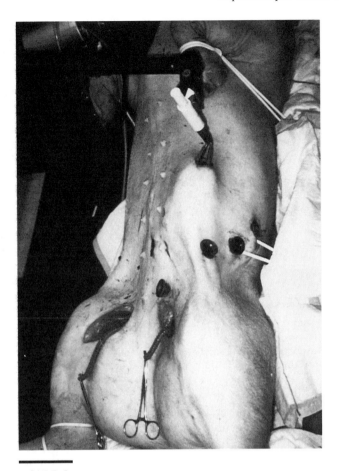

FIGURE 1.

This photograph demonstrates the view of the porcine model of Dion and Gracia. Note the supine position of the subject for an anterolateral retroperitoneal approach to the aorta, which allows simultaneous proximal control at all times with exposure of the groins for tunneling of the prosthesis and distal anastomosis.

sewn intraluminally while bleeding as in conventional repair. The anastomosis was constructed in end-to-end fashion by suturing from within the aorta and incorporating an intact posterior wall to reproduce the open technique of endo-aneurysmorraphy. All anastomoses were constructed with standard monofilament 4–0 prolene suture using curved vascular needles in continuous fashion.

The results demonstrated reproducible construction of an aortobifemoral bypass in less than four hours (Fig 2). Blood loss never exceeded 550 mL, with bleeding most commonly occurring when

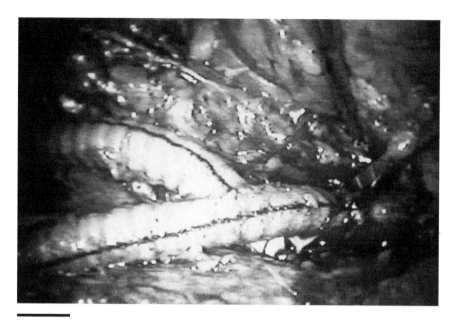

FIGURE 2.
This photograph demonstrates the completed aortoprosthetic anastamosis in the porcine model of Dion and Gracia. This is completed in end-to-end fashion.

the aorta was opened and flushed, and on occasion from the over-sewn aortoiliac stump after the limbs of the grafts were opened. This was corrected with additional suture as necessary. In these early models, the totally laparoscopic aortic anastomosis did not take more than 60 minutes to perform. The magnification afforded by a well-placed laparoscope allowed for an excellent view for meticulous completion of the anastomosis. No operative mortality was encountered in this series, or in the previous, which together account for 34 consecutive totally laparoscopic aortobifemoral bypasses.

In these experiments, piglets were selected because of their reproducibility and their comparable anatomy in the retroperitoneal aorta and surrounding structures to the human. The abdominal wall of the piglet is composed of the same muscles as is in humans,[11] and it was thought that this animal model allowed performance of an aortobifemoral bypass in conditions similar to those encountered in humans. However, the actual end organs, the human aorta and iliac arteries, are considerably different than those of the porcine model. The actual size of the vessels is different. The Yorkshire-cross piglet, despite its enormous size (75–80 kg), has an aorta that typically measures 7–8 mm in diameter. The aortic prosthesis is constructed from grafts of 6 mm in diameter and sewn to each other in end-to-side fashion to form an appropriate bifurcated prosthesis for aortobifemoral bypass. However, based on our clinical experience, the larger human aorta (16 mm diameter) has proven technically easier to work with because of its size, which facilitates many of the maneuvers used in laparoscopic suturing in a confined space such as the retroperitoneum.

The porcine vessels also have no atheromata present within them. The available instrumentation and laparoscopic suture techniques may not prove feasible in the face of calcified atheromatous plaque. After having completed much of the previously referenced laboratory work, the authors applied laparoscopic instrumentation in standard open aortoprosthetic anastomosis for occlusive disease. This application of the instrumentation allowed for evaluation in the presence of atheromata, and fortunately, no major limitations were identified. The tactile feedback critical to a surgeon working with instruments is just as palpable with the laparoscopic tools as is experienced with open tools. Assessment of the calcified plaque with the needle tip to determine how and where to place it was comparable between open and laparoscopic needle drivers.

The anterolateral retroperitoneal approach possesses numerous advantages over both the transabdominal and lateral approach. Although more difficult than the complete lateral approach, the surgeon and assistant work in the same fashion as if the abdomen were opened. The large size of this animal model (Yorkshire piglets, 75–80 kg) also makes comparison with human surgery more realistic because the instruments used in these experiments were the same as used for humans. Laparoscopic occlusive clamps, scalpel holders, potz scissors (Laborie Surgical Ltd), all early in design, were limited, but available.

The animal model also falls short in re-creating the aortic aneurysm. In addition, the commonplace destruction of the posterior wall of the aorta in aneurysmal disease is also not available in the non-atheromatous porcine aorta. However, aside from this it does serve to re-create the working environment around the aorta, e.g., control bleeding of the lumbar arteries and suturing from within the aorta using the intact posterior wall, as required for aneurysm repair in the human.

TRANSITION TO HUMAN CLINICAL EXPERIENCE

Consistent exposure and anastomosis in the laboratory animal model proved achievable without excessive operative blood loss, time, or mortality. Two major areas of concern remained prior to using this technique in the operating room. The first was whether to proceed with a gasless technique, as had proven successful in the laboratory, or to proceed with insufflation in patients to enlarge the working space. If insufflation were used, what are the risks of gas embolism? The second major area of concern was how the animal model applied to the human in terms of port placement and the actual hands-on comparison of the anatomy. Despite all the anatomical similarities, was the procedure from the animal model directly applicable in the human?

The potential for gas embolism was evaluated by Dion.[14] Since carbon dioxide embolization during laparoscopy is a recognized and potentially lethal complication,[15, 16] the potential for pulmonary embolization following major venous laceration was evaluated under laparoscopic conditions. A model with anesthetized dogs and hemodynamic monitoring via an arterial line and Swan-Ganz catheter was evaluated under carbon dioxide pneumoperitoneum. Transesophageal echocardiography was used to evaluate the status and amount of embolism within the heart chambers. Euvolemic dogs were submitted to a 1-cm longitudinal incision made into the vena cava while maintaining a carbon dioxide pneumoperitoneum with pressures between 12 and 15 mmHg. No gas embolism was seen in 82% of the cases after exposure of the venotomies to the pneumoperitoneum, and only 18% had gas bubbles visible in the right heart cavities by transesophageal echocardiography. In contrast, direct intravenous bolus injection of only 15 mL of carbon dioxide led to visualization of many more gas bubbles in the right heart cavities. Massive injections intravenously of CO_2 (>300 cc) led to the appearance of gas bubbles in the left heart cavities and death.

These experiments also demonstrated that detection of gas embolism is more precise using the transesophageal echocardiography probe than relying on elevation of pulmonary artery pressure. A bolus of 15 cc of CO_2 was visualized easily without concomitant elevation of pulmonary artery pressure. The routine use of transesophageal echocardiography has not been clinically encouraged since in clinical practice very few episodes of gas embolism have been reported. In three studies, the incidence of gas embolism was respectively one in 63,845 patients, 15 in 113,253 patients, and eight in 50,247 patients.[17] As a result of these studies, it was thought that it would be safe to proceed under routine pneumoperitoneum if necessary and/or helpful.

The second area of concern was the applicability of the animal model to the human anatomy. The best way to evaluate this was to proceed in the human cadaver laboratory. A series of experiences were collected by re-creating the retroperitoneal working space, normally a potential space. The natural tissue planes lend themselves to ready dissection to create an actual space that had not previously existed. What was learned proved valuable in terms of being able to re-create the working space by application of the acquired experience from the animal model. Blunt dissection proved difficult, but application of balloon technology (General Surgical Innovations, Cupertino, Ca) allowed rapid and reproducible dissection and conversion of this retroperitoneal space from potential to actual. Carbon dioxide pneumoretroperitoneum was used with pressures of 12–14 mmHg to maintain the space, allowing placement of other working trocars for dissection, retraction, occlusion of the aorta, and creation of the retroperitoneal tunnels in which to place the vascular prosthetic graft. The actual placement sites for all the required trocars were then sorted out.

HUMAN CLINICAL EXPERIENCE

As was previously noted, the first human aortic vascular experience was successfully carried out by Dion.[1] Ischemic rest pain due to aortoiliac occlusive inflow disease developed in a 63-year-old man with a history of myocardial infarction; he underwent a laparoscopically-assisted aortobifemoral bypass graft. The patient experienced neither cardiac nor pulmonary complications and was able to take deep breaths and move without discomfort. Less depression of pulmonary function following laparoscopy was anticipated based on experience with laparoscopic cholycystectomy,[18] but could not be assumed.

This initial experience seemed very encouraging, and as a result, four additional such procedures were reported.[7] The only intraoperative complication was a small-bowel perforation due to retraction difficulties in this transperitoneal route. Postoperatively, patients felt less pain and were able to cough more effectively and walk more easily. There were no postoperative complications.

In a second series, reported by Berens and Herde,[8] a variety of procedures included one left iliofemoral bypass, one aortobifemoral bypass, one right iliofemoral bypass, and one aortoiliac endarterectomy. The two iliac patients were ambulating early and discharged in 24 hours. The aortic patients were taking a diet at 48 hours postoperatively and discharged on the third day without any complications. The technique involved transperitoneal laparoscopic abdominal dissection and graft insertion using an abdominal wall lift device (Origin Medsystems, Menlo Park, Ca).

There were several concerns addressed in this report. A gasless laparoscopic-assisted approach was selected to mimic the risk of gas embolism and the technical difficulty of a totally laparoscopic vascular anastomosis. Paramidline incisions of 4 cm in length were made to facilitate insertion of conventional instrumentation for construction of hemostatic suture lines. Nonetheless, this experience reinforced the earlier experience of Dion that the postoperative course of the patients with a laparoscopic-assisted aortobifemoral bypass graft was highlighted by a more rapid recovery of the patients. Both early approaches used a transperitoneal route, whereas Dion used gas insufflation for the working space and Berets used abdominal wall suspension. The two initial reports noted the difficulties in retraction of intraabdominal organs, rendering aortic dissection and end-to-side aortoprosthetic anastomosis rather tedious.

The authors were subsequently influenced to pursue the retroperitoneal approach in the animal models.[13] There were also advantages to a totally laparoscopic approach as opposed to laparoscopic-assisted. Experienced laparoscopists recognize that "lap-assisted" or "mini-lap" procedures are potentially very difficult, particularly in patients in whom the abdominal wall is very thick and the intraperitoneal fatty mass increases, rendering retraction and exposure increasingly difficult. A totally laparoscopic retroperitoneal approach had the potential to solve many of the early problems.

As a result of our laboratory experiences[13, 19–22] and the evaluation of a retroperitoneal approach to completely laparoscopic aortobifemoral bypass in human cadavers, we began our clinical experience in March of 1995. A total of seven patients have undergone successful aortoiliac bypass for occlusive disease with either aortobifemoral bypass graft (five patients) or iliofemoral graft (two patients). They ranged in age from 62 to 71 years old, and six were men. The indications for surgery were rest pain in one (ankle-brachial index [ABI] <0.20) and severe claudication in six (ABI <0.60). Patients underwent appropriate preoperative cardiopulmonary evaluation to be certain they were candidates for the standard open approach. All patients were given the option of interventional procedures, but were not considered as ideal candidates for such treatment based on the extent and distribution of the arteriosclerotic disease on arteriography. In one case, a patient had undergone successful bilateral common iliac artery stent placement for isolated stenosis, which recurred in less than 18 months with re-current symptoms.

We began with a right iliofemoral bypass graft for a completely occluded right external iliac artery. The application of the retro-peritoneal dissection established a satisfactory working space with gas insufflation and the end-to-end anastomosis was constructed without difficulty. This patient required minimal analgesics and was discharged from the hospital in 48 hours. In the second case we used a gasless space with abdominal wall suspension. We ex-perienced difficulties in maintaining the working space and expo-sure required for dissection and proximal anastomosis of the aor-tobifemoral graft, resulting in a lengthy operation of approximately 12 hours. Cross-clamp time approached 240 minutes. Compartment syndromes with myoglobinuria developed that were readily iden-tified and treated, but contributed to a lengthier hospital stay.

While valuable experience was gained from these first two cases, the advantages of working under insufflation were not eas-ily dismissed. If exposure could be consistently maintained with insufflation, adaptation of basic vascular instrumentation should allow for vascular anastomoses to be constructed in this totally laparoscopic environment. For these reasons we began to work with insufflation in all subsequent cases.

With the second aortic case, we experience improved visibil-ity and exposure under insufflation (Fig 3), yet surgical time was still long at approximately 10 hours. Aortic cross-clamp time, how-ever, dropped to 70 minutes. The patient required minimal anal-gesics postoperatively, there was no subcutaneous emphysema, and the patient ambulated and started a diet within 48 hours of surgery. Although he could have been discharged in 72 hours, he was observed for an additional 24 hours, more in line with the re-covery expected for MIS procedures. The surgical time was still lengthy, but many of the early applications of laparoscopy to stan-dard gastrointestinal procedures were commonly several hours. Technology did improve the ability to carry out laborious tasks in shorter times. Ultimately, surgical experience with laparoscopy in the working space, the anatomy, and the currently available tech-nology have a significant impact on reducing surgery times. For laparoscopy to be successful for aortobifemoral or iliofemoral by-pass grafting, further evolution of techniques is necessary and op-erative times need to decrease.

Much of this evolution occurred in the next several cases. Gas insufflation was continued, as it had proved to be superior in pro-ducing the best working space and did not pose difficulties with

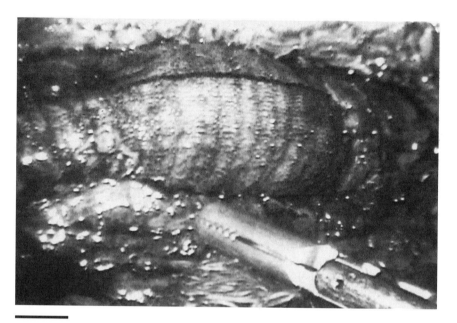

FIGURE 3.

This is a photograph of the completed end-to-end aortoprosthetic anastomosis completed in the clinical series of Dion and Gracia. In this case, standard CO_2 gas insufflation at 12–15 mmHg is used in place of abdominal wall suspension.

suction or the other tasks associated with vascular surgery. Significant reduction in overall surgical times was achieved with the last two AFBs performed within 5–6 hours with cross-clamp times between 80 and 120 minutes, depending on how much work was required in the groins at the femoral or profunda femoris vessels. Hospital stays averaged 4 to 5 days, but all patients could have been discharged sooner. There was only one conversion from the totally laparoscopic approach, which occurred in one female who sustained a disruption of a calcified plaque by the aortic clamp, resulting in immediate occlusion. A mini-laparotomy of 4 to 5 cm was performed to explore the anastomosis and endarterectomize the site of cross-clamping. With a retroperitoneal approach, small renal vein retractors were inserted behind a retroperitoneal apron to readily expose the area without interference from tenuous bowel retraction. All anastomoses were accomplished in end-to-end fashion, with the exception of the final end-to-side iliofemoral anastomosis required to preserve the patent internal iliac. Intracorporeal laparoscopic suturing with continuous monofilament suture was used in all cases.

The prolonged operative time required for these cases was primarily attributed to careful creation of the retroperitoneal cavity, key to successful completion of the bypass. In contrast, the aortic anastomosis was generally completed within 50 to 60 minutes. Much of the decreases in surgical time were due to increased familiarity with the retroperitoneal anatomy as seen laparoscopically. For example, in the last two aortic cases, the time required to establish the retroperitoneal work space and complete the dissection was decreased from over 4 hours to less than 2 hours.

ABDOMINAL AORTIC ANEURYSMS

The surgical treatment for abdominal aortic aneurysm has involved the placement of a graft in the involved areas. Mortality rates remained high until 1966, when Creech reported on the technique of endo-aneurysmorrhaphy.[23] Continued improvements in modern anesthetic techniques and critical care have contributed to the decreased mortality rates of 2% to 4%.[24]

The percutaneous placement of endoluminal stent-grafts is directed at avoiding the morbidity and mortality associated with major abdominal surgery. However, endovascular grafts require high skill for implantation[25] and are subject to unique complications themselves, although technical success is achieved in the majority of cases. May et al. report a vascular complication rate of 10% for a tube graft, which rises to 43% for a bifurcated endovascular graft.[26] In another trial with 46 patients, Moore and Rutherford[27] report contrast enhancement outside the graft but within the aneurysmal sac in 17 grafts (44%), of which 9 (51%) resolved spontaneously. Hospital stay varied between 1 and 14 days.[28, 29] Uncontrolled lumbar vessels have also raised concern regarding continued aneurysmal growth.

The surgical approach to infrarenal aortic aneurysm requires a lengthy xipho-pubic incision associated with considerable postoperative pain. Postoperative care requires an expensive critical care stay and an additional 5 to 7 days in the hospital. As applied to abdominal aortic aneurysm repair, the MIS techniques used with other abdominal laparoscopic procedures may yield similar advantages.

A porcine model to evaluate laparoscopic aortic aneurysm repair was reported by Chen et al.[28] In these experiments, there were 15 successful graft insertions in 21 pigs undergoing transabdominal dissection of the aorta. Six were unsuccessful because of technical, anatomical, or bleeding difficulties. Two grafts were attempted retroperitoneally, and only one was successful due to a tear in the peritoneum of the other. Other complications noted included injuries to bladder, ureter, renal vein, inferior vena cava, aorta, and lumbar vessel. However, as experience was gained, operative time decreased from 6 to less than 2 hours with concomitant reduction in estimated blood loss from 1,000 mL to less than 150 mL.

Chen and co-workers used an endoluminal graft inserted by aortotomy and secured in place by extraluminal umbilical tapes. In our model,[13] we attempted to reproduce the endo-aneurysmhorrhaphy technique of suturing a graft in place with an intact back wall and intraluminal control of lumbar vessels. However, both animal experiences lack aneurysmal mass or mural calcification. Without this mass the dissection is simpler, and without the calcification there is minimal risk of distal embolization.

This work primarily has resulted in the successful completion of laparoscopic-assisted repair of infrarenal abdominal aortic aneurysm in humans by Chen and colleagues.[29] A 62-year-old man underwent successful repair of an asymptomatic 6 cm aortic abdominal aneurysm. This first case was completed with ten trocars and a 10 cm mini-laparotomy. Total operative time was 4 hours and estimated blood loss was 1,000 mL. The approach was transabdominal and bowel retraction was facilitated by a "fish" retractor modified for the special task. They reported decreased volume requirements with early mobilization of fluids, a quicker return of bowel function, and an earlier discharge on postoperative day 6. In subsequent cases, Chen and co-workers have since simplified the approach, reducing the number of trocars to six (Chen, personal communication). This work contributes to establish the feasibility of laparoscopic aortic surgery, whether totally laparoscopic or laparoscopic-assisted.

A third approach to the treatment of abdominal aortic aneurysm by MIS consists of a combined endovascular and laparoscopic approach. This may help to solve many of the challenging problems encountered during the performance of one of these two described techniques. However, this new approach has yet to be described.

CONCLUSIONS

We think that laparoscopic aortic surgery is feasible and the further development of minimal access vascular aortoiliac surgery should be based on established principles.[30] The technique has been shown to be feasible in the laboratory,[11, 13, 19-22] and has been performed on a few well-selected patients.[31] The totally laparo-scopic approach to the aortoiliac segment in our experience appears to be more appealing than a laparoscopic-assisted method using an 8 to 10 cm incision. Thus far, it has been safely performed with current "off-the-shelf" instrumentation.

To promote the safety, efficacy, reproducibility, and ability to teach the procedures, many areas require improvement. Clearly, in-strument design is critical. Standard vascular instruments need to be adapted to work laparoscopically. Occlusion devices need to be designed or adapted to work laparoscopically and may incorporate external handles or detachable intracorporeal clamps (e.g., bull dogs). Technology will improve our ability to provide rapid and consistent exposure and maintenance of the retroperitonial space. The issue of a gas or gasless approach is certainly not resolved. The former allows for better exposure because of the three-dimensional push of the gas under pressure. However, a gasless approach al-lows unique instrumentation and the ability to apply more suction. The risk of gas embolism has been well studied by Dion et al.,[14] but a combination of the two approaches (gas and gasless) may be possible.

Finally, the anastomosis will require instrumentation that pro-vides consistent construction of a safe and durable anastomosis. A number of technologies are under evaluation for this purpose. Cur-rent experience with laparoscopy among vascular surgeons is ex-tremely variable. Over the next several years, however, experience should be more uniform as many of tomorrow's vascular surgeons will have had laparoscopic training and experience in gastrointes-tinal surgery. Also, understanding the importance of the need for increased skills and experience in laparoscopy will allow laparo-scopic suturing to be more prevalent.

Laparoscopic vascular surgery of the infrarenal aortoiliac seg-ment has extraordinary potential and differs from conventional re-construction only by the approach. The long-term results are there-fore expected to be similar. Performing laparoscopic surgery for oc-clusive disease is presently easier for abdominal aortic aneurysms, but ongoing experience supports continued investigation and de-velopment of these techniques. Laparoscopic aortoiliac surgery re-mains in the feasibility state, at present, but the initial favorable experience supports plans now in progress for a multicenter trial of laparoscopic aortobifemoral bypass.

REFERENCES

1. Brewster DC: Current controversies in the management of aortoiliac occlusive disease. *J Vasc Surg* 25:365–379, 1997.

2. Périssat J, Collet D, Belliard R: Traitement laparoscopique par lithotripsie intra-corporelle suivi de cholécystostomie ou de cholécystectomie. *Chirurgie* 116:243–247, 1990.

3. Svenberg T: Pathophysiology of pneumoperitoneum, in Ballantyne GH, Leahy PF, Modlin IM (eds): *Laparoscopic Surgery.* Montreal, WB Saunders, 1994, pp 61–68.

4. Peters JH, Ortega A, Lehnerd SL, et al: The physiology of laparoscopic surgery: Pulmonary function after laparoscopic cholecystectomy. *Surg Laparosc Endosc* 3:370–374, 1993.

5. Poulin EC, Mamazza J, Breton G, et al: Evaluation of pulmonary function in laparoscopic cholecystectomy. *Surg Laparosc Endosc* 2:292–296, 1993.

6. Dion YM, Katkhouda N, Rouleau C, et al: Laparoscopy-assisted aortobifemoral bypass. *Surg Laparosc Endosc* 3:425–429, 1993.

7. Dion YM, Rouleau C, Aucoin A: Laparoscopy-assisted aortobifemoral bypass. *Surg Endosc* 8:438, 1994.

8. Berens E, Herde JR: Laparoscopic vascular surgery: Four case reports. *J Vasc Surg* 22:73–79, 1995.

9. Ahn SS, Clem MF, Braithwaite BD, et al: Laparoscopic aortofemoral bypass, initial experience in an animal model. *Ann Surg* 5:677–683, 1995.

10. Jones DB, Thompson RW, Soper NJ, et al: Development and comparison of transperitoneal and retroperitoneal approaches to laparoscopic-assisted aortofemoral bypass in a porcine model. *J Vasc Surg* 23:466–471, 1996.

11. Dion YM, Chin AK, Thompson TA: Experimental laparoscopic aortobifemoral bypass. *Surg Endosc* 9:894–897, 1995.

12. Schumaker HB: Midline extraperitoneal exposure of the abdominal aorta and the iliac arteries. *Surg Gynecol Obstet* 135:791–792, 1972.

13. Dion YM, Gracia CR: Experimental laparoscopic aortic aneurysm resection and aortobifemoral bypass. *Surg Laparosc Endosc* 6:184–190, 1996.

14. Dion YM, Levesque C, Doillon CJ: Experimental carbon dioxide pulmonary embolization after vena cava laceration under pneumoperitoneum. *Surg Endosc* 9:1065–1069, 1995.

15. Chui PT, Gin T, Oh TE: Anaesthesia for laparoscopic general surgery. *Anaesth Intensive Care* 21:163–171, 1993.

16. McQuaide JR: Air embolism during peritoneoscopy. *S Afr Med J* 46:422–423, 1972.

17. De Plaizer RMH, Jones ISC: Non-fatal carbon dioxide embolism during laparoscopy. *Anaesth Intensive Care* 17:359–361, 1989.

18. Rademaker BM, Ringers J, Odoom JA, et al: Pulmonary function and stress response after laparoscopic cholycystectomy: Comparison with subcostal incision and influence of thoracic epidural analgesia. *Anesth Analg* 75:381–385, 1992.

19. Dion YM, Gaillard F, Demalsy JC, et al: Experimental laparoscopic aor-

tobifemoral bypass for occlusive aortoiliac disease. *Can J Surg* 39:451–455, 1996.

20. Dion YM, Gracia CR, Demalsy JC, et al: Laparoscopic aortic surgery: animal and human clinical evaluation. *Minimally Invasive Therapy* 4:40, 1995.

21. Dion YM, Gracia CR: A reproducible animal model for laparoscopic retroperitoneal aortobifemoral bypass in aortoiliac occlusive disease. *Surg Endosc* 10:270, 1996.

22. Dion YM, Gracia CR, Demalsy JC, et al: Laparoscopic and laparoscopy-assisted aortoiliac surgery: Animal and clinical evaluation. *J Endocvasc Surg* 3:114, 1996.

23. Creech Jr O: Endo-aneurysmorrhaphy and treatment of aortic aneurysm. *Ann Surg* 164:936–946, 1966.

24. Cambria RP, Brewster DC, Abbott WM, et al: Transperitoneal vs. retroperitoneal approach for aortic reconstruction: A randomized prospective study. *J Vasc Surg* 11:314–325, 1990.

25. Veith FJ, Marin ML: Endovascular surgery and its effect on the relationship between vascular surgery and radiology. *J Endovasc Surg* 2:1–7, 1995.

26. May J, White JH, Yu W, et al: Results of endoluminal grafting of abdominal aortic aneurysms are dependent on aneurysm morphology. *Ann Vasc Surg* 10:254–261, 1996.

27. Moore WS, Rutherford RB: Transfemoral endovascular repair of abdominal aortic aneurysm: Results of the North American EVT phase I trial. *J Vasc Surg* 23:543–552, 1996.

28. Chen HM, Murphy EA, Levison J, et al: Laparoscopic aortic replacement in the porcine model: A feasibility study in preparation for laparoscopically assisted abdominal aortic aneurysm repair in humans. *J Am Coll Surg* 183:126–132, 1996.

29. Chen HM, Murphy EA, Halpern V, et al: Laparoscopic-assisted abdominal aortic aneurysm repair. *Surg Endosc* 9:905–907, 1995.

30. Schrock TR: The endosurgery evolution: No place for sacred cows. *Surg Endosc* 6:163–168, 1992.

31. Dion YM, Gracia CR, Demalsy JC: Laparoscopic aortic surgery. *J Vasc Surg* 23:539, 1995.

CHAPTER 10

Management of Mycotic Aneurysms

Dennis F. Bandyk, M.D.
Professor of Surgery; Director, Division of Vascular Surgery; The
University of South Florida College of Medicine, Division of Vascular
Surgery, Tampa, Florida

Infection involving the peripheral arteries was among the first vascular lesions surgeons managed. When patients presented with the triad of a febrile illness, pulsatile mass, and positive blood culture results, procedures consisting of arterial ligation, and, if feasible, excision, or limb amputation were performed to deal with a spontaneous mycotic aneurysm or arterial bleeding from a contaminated traumatic wound. The term "mycotic" orginated from Osler, who described in his Gulstonian lectures of 1885 the clinical manifestations and sequelae of aortic and peripheral artery infections that resulted from bacterial endocarditis.[1] Abscesses involving artery walls had been described earlier in the 19th century, but Osler was the first to recognize the propensity of bacterial vegetations on the aortic valves to embolize and infect remote arteries. Antibiotic treatment of endocarditis, microbiologic and echocardiographic diagnostic techniques, and replacement of infected cardiac valves have markedly reduced the incidence of septic embolic complications.

The term "mycotic aneurysm" denotes the invasion and disruption of the arterial wall by microorganisms. These aneurysms are rare; vascular referral centers encounter this entity only ten to 20 times per decade. Infected arterial aneurysms are identified in 0.4% of postmortem examinations and are a presenting sign in 3% of patients with abdominal aortic aneurysm.[2–4] Although mycotic aneurysms can occur anywhere in the arterial tree, the majority develop in the thoracic and abdominal aorta. Diagnosis and successful eradication of an infectious process involving the aorta remains among the most challenging problems in vascular surgery. Delays in recognition and treatment significantly increase morbidity due to sepsis, artery wall erosion into adjacent organs, and hemorrhage associated with rupture. Infected aneurysms can occur spontaneously as a result of remote infection (endocarditis, hematogenous seeding), following cannulation of arteries and veins for drug administration, pressure monitoring, diagnostic studies, and after therapeutic endovascular procedures (transluminal angioplasty, atherectomy, stent or vena cava filter placement). The invasive nature of modern medicine and, unfortunately, persistent drug/substance abuse have produced a resurgence of arterial infections from penetrating injuries, which introduces contamination at the vessel wall puncture site or in an adjacent hematoma. The incidence of mycotic aneurysm associated with bacterial endocarditis or following endovascular procedures is uncommon (less than 1%), but conditions such as chronic illness, malnutrition, and impaired immune function appear to increase its occurrence.

CLASSIFICATION

Mycotic aneurysms can be classified based on the mechanisms by which infecting organisms invade the vessel wall, preexisting status of the arterial segment, and anatomic site.[5, 6] The term mycotic aneurysm was used by Osler to denote any vascular infection caused by microorganisms, including fungal infections. In present-day vascular surgery, the term mycotic aneurysm is used in a broader sense to encompass both false or pseudoaneurysms caused by arterial infection as well as true aneurysms that have become secondarily infected. A diseased aorta with atherosclerotic plaque and mural thrombus is more susceptible to colonization from bacteremia. Gram-positive bacteria, such as staphylococci and streptococci, can be trapped within plaque or thrombus, infecting the adjacent diseased artery wall, and produce local suppuration followed by loss of wall tensile strength. These lesions are fulminant infections, typically associated with fever, septicemia, acute aneurysm expansion, or rupture; and are distinct from the more common clinical scenario of culture-positive aneurysm sac contents in a patient without local or systemic signs of infection.

Mycotic aneurysms can develop by one of three mechanisms: direct extension of an adjacent suppurative focus (extravascular), bacterial colonization of diseased arterial segments (intravascular), and septic emboli as a result of endocarditis (embolomycotic) or septicemia (known or unknown source) with organisms entering the vessel wall at sites of damaged endothelium or the vasa vasorum (cryptogenic). The syphilitic aneurysm is a classic cryptogenic mycotic aneurysm and accounted for 50% of all aneurysms in the pre-antibiotic era usually affecting the ascending aorta. Aortic stump sepsis is a rare and unique vascular lesion, produced by residual artery wall infection after excision of an infected aortic graft or aneurysm, and ligation of the aorta.

PATHOPHYSIOLOGY AND ANATOMICAL DISTRIBUTION

No artery is immune to the development of infection. There is considerable experimental evidence to indicate bacteremia alone rarely causes infection in a "normal" artery, although important exceptions include particulate embolism from a proximal septic focus and arteritis produced by syphilis or tuberculosis, and arterial invasion by *Salmonella* species. Risk of infection increases at sites of atherosclerotic lesions, in particular aneurysms, and at sites of iatrogenic, accidental, or self-induced penetrating arterial trauma. Direct arterial trauma is the prevalent etiologic factor for mycotic aneurysms diagnosed and treated in clinical practice. A common form involves infection of a surgically created arteriovenous fistula for chronic hemodialysis. Inoculation of the vessel wall can occur at the time of an injury or operative manipulation, from a contiguous septic process via periarterial lymphatics or vasa vasorum, or by embolism of septic microemboli to arterial branch points or arterial vasa vasorum. Intercurrent bacteremia from any source can result in the trapping of microorganisms in any intimal defect, especially vessels with atherosclerotic plaque and mural thrombus. Whether an infection becomes established depends on both the quantity and virulence of the pathogens as well as host resistance factors.

Early diagnosis and antibiotic treatment of bacterial endocarditis and syphilis have altered the anatomical distribution of mycotic aneurysms. The classic luetic thoracic aortic aneurysm is now rarely seen in the western world, whereas it used to be responsible for one half of all aneurysms. In the pre-antibiotic era, the proportion of aortic to peripheral mycotic aneurysms was relatively high. Infection frequently occurred at the site of preexisting arterial disease (congenital lesion, atherosclerotic aneurysm) or developed as a consequence of untreated endocarditis. While embolomycotic aneurysms still occur, the majority of mycotic aneurysms are now extravascular or intravascular in origin, the most frequent being the result of direct trauma (drug abuse, endovascular procedures) and concomitant bacterial contamination. Collected series of mycotic aneurysms indicate the femoral artery is the prevalent location, fol-

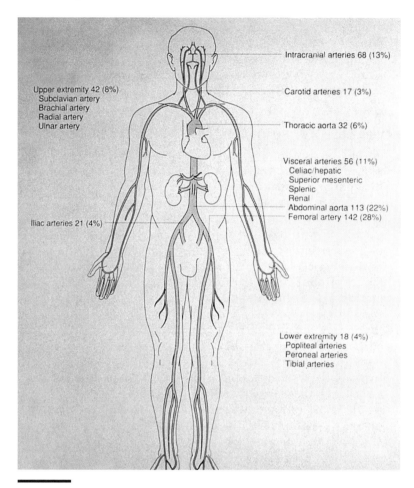

Intracranial arteries 68 (13%)

Carotid arteries 17 (3%)

Upper extremity 42 (8%)
Subclavian artery
Brachial artery
Radial artery
Ulnar artery

Thoracic aorta 32 (6%)

Visceral arteries 56 (11%)
Celiac/hepatic
Superior mesenteric
Splenic
Renal
Abdominal aorta 113 (22%)
Femoral artery 142 (28%)

Iliac arteries 21 (4%)

Lower extremity 18 (4%)
Popliteal arteries
Peroneal arteries
Tibial arteries

FIGURE 1.

Anatomical distribution of 510 mycotic aneurysms from collected series.

lowed by the abdominal aorta and visceral vessels[2–9] (Fig 1). Mycotic aortic aneurysms tend to be saccular and develop in the transverse aortic arch or in the thoracoabdominal aorta especially in the region posterior to the origin of the visceral (celiac, superior mesenteric, renal) arteries.

CLINICAL MANIFESTATIONS

Presenting symptoms and signs of arterial infection are varied and often subtle. The triad of localized pain, a pulsatile mass, and fever suggests the presence of an infected arterial aneurysm. A history of bacterial endocarditis, other sources of septicemia (urosepsis, pneumonia, infected vascular catheters, septic thrombophlebitis, cellulitis), osteomyelitis of the spine, or recent penetrating trauma are important risk factors. No source of infection can be identified in approximately one-quarter of patients. When located in the extremities, the mycotic aneurysm can be palpated in most patients (over 80%). Petechial skin lesions and septic arthritis can occur due to peripheral embolism, and a systolic bruit may be present over the lesion. If the infectious process is deeply situated in the abdomen or thorax, the aneurysm is not palpable and clinical presentation is a fever of unknown origin (FUO). Abdominal pain was present in only 35% of patients with infected abdominal aortic aneurysms with the aneurysm palpable in one-half of cases. Myalgias, arthralgias, episodes of fever and chills, or progressive weakness typically are present for weeks before the diagnosis of mycotic aneurysm is made. Intracerebral mycotic aneurysms present with lateralizing hemispheric deficits secondary to rupture, or lethargy and confusion due to abscess formation.

Most patients (over 90%) have one or multiple risk factors for the development of mycotic aneurysms; the most common entities are arterial trauma, depressed immune function (corticosteroid administration, chronic renal failure, malignancy, chemotherapy), and concurrent sepsis or bacterial endocarditis. One quarter of patients with mycotic aneurysms have documented cellular or humoral immunodeficiency.[8, 9] The rarity of mycotic aneurysms in the absence of obvious risk factors attests to the immunity of the normal artery wall to invasive bacterial infection. Salmonellal septicemia usually occurs in elderly patients with predisposing factors such as autoimmune diseases, diabetes, and corticosteroid or immunosuppressive medication.

The ultimate manifestation of arterial infection, regardless of location, is wall weakening or disruption, leading to aneurysm formation, contained rupture, or hemorrhage. Artery wall infections are complex processes involving tissue destruction from activation of host defenses by the microorganisms as well as bacterial by-products of metabolism. The inflammatory response to infection disrupts wall anatomy and decreases tensile strength. With the formation of an aneurysm or development of a contained rupture, bacteria-laden thrombus is deposited, forming a septic nidus thereby permitting continuous bacteria shedding and bacteremia. Less virulent pathogens, such as *Staphylococcus epidermidis* and other coagulase-negative staphylococci have a limited capacity to produce an invasive vascular infection and, in general, require the presence of a foreign body (intravascular catheter, prosthetic graft) to sustain the infectious process.

BACTERIOLOGY

Although virtually any organism can infect the vascular system, *S. aureus* is the prevalent pathogen of mycotic aneurysms and infected aortic aneurysms (Table 1). Over the past two decades, the microbiology of mycotic aneurysms has changed with an increased frequency of infections caused by gram-negative organisms, such as *Escherichia coli, Pseudomonas* sp., *Klebsiella* sp., *Enterobacter* sp., and *Proteus* sp. and fungi *(Candida, Aspergillus)*. Aneurysms infected with gram-negative organisms have an increased rupture rate

---

TABLE 1.

Bacteriology of Mycotic Aneurysms

	Incidence from Collected Series (%)	
Microorganism	**Mycotic Aneurysm**	**Infected AAA**
Streptococcus sp.	10	20
Staphylococcus aureus	30	40
Staphylococcus epidermidis	5	10–15
Salmonella sp.	20	<1
Pseudomonas sp.	10	2
Escherichia coli	10	5
Proteus sp.	4	2
Klebsiella sp.	3	2
Enterobacter sp.	3	1
Enterococcus group	2	<1
Serratia sp.	3	2
Candida sp.	2	2
Mycobacterium tuberculosis	1	—
Other species	5–10	5–10
Bacteroides fragilis		
Arizona hinshawii		
Citrobacter freundii		
Campylobacter fetus		
Listeria monocytogenes		
Culture negative	10–15	—

Abbreviation: AAA, abdominal aortic aneurysm

(80%) compared to infections due to gram-positive organisms (10%). Infections due to *Pseudomonas* sp. are particularly virulent because of the organisms' ability to produce destructive endotoxins (elastase, alkaline protease) that act against elastin and collagen in artery and vein graft walls to compromise structural integrity. Coagulase-positive staphylococci and streptococci sp. also produce lysins that are hemolytic and result in cell necrosis and necrosis of mobilized leukocytes. Infections produced by *S. aureus* and gram-negative bacteria involve invasion of tissue and are associated with a high concentration of bacteria (10^5 to 10^7 colony-forming units [CFU]). Most patients with fungal vascular infections are either immunosuppressed or have established fungal infections elsewhere. Swabs of tissue surfaces, fluid, and perigraft exudate imprinted on agar media can be associated with significant sampling error if low (less than 10^4 CFUs) numbers of bacteria are present. Microbiologic sampling error results in negative culture results in up to one-quarter of patients with mycotic aneurysms.[2, 4, 7, 9, 10–12]

Salmonella sp are the infecting pathogen of most intravascular mycotic aneurysms, typically involving the thoracic or abdominal aorta, and on occasion the femoral artery. Contaminated water, poultry, and meat products are the most important sources of these gram-negative, flagellated bacteria, which have a predilection for diseased arterial walls. The portal of entry is the gastrointestinal tract and the biliary tree, with the subsequent clinical course determined by extent of mucosal invasion, serotype involved, and host resistance. Children and adults with lymphoproliferative disorders or sickle cell anemia are particularly vulnerable to develop salmonellal bacteremia and extravascular metastatic sites of infection (osteomyelitis of lumbar vertebrae, paravertebral abscesses, meningitis). There are more than 2,200 serotypes, but *S. cholerae-suis, S. typhimurium,* and *S. enteritidis* account for two-thirds of the arterial infections.

DIAGNOSTIC MODALITIES

Prompt diagnosis and treatment of infected aneurysms are essential to avoid complications (septic emboli, rupture) and fatal outcomes. Blood culture results are positive in 50% to 75% of patients with mycotic infections. Leukocytosis and increased erythrocyte sedimentation rate are common but nonspecific findings in patients with vascular infections and fever.

Vascular imaging is a vital component of the evaluation of patients with suspected or proven vascular infection. Both anatomical and functional diagnostic imaging techniques may be necessary to confirm the presence of infection, plan management, and assess operative sites for residual or recurrent infection.

Anatomical imaging techniques
Ultrasonography
Computed tomography (CT)
Magnetic resonance imaging/angiography (MRI/MRA)
Digital subtraction/conventional contrast arteriography

Functional imaging techniques
^{99m}Tc-hexametazime—labeled leukocytes
^{111}In-labeled leukocyte scan
^{111}In-labeled immunoglobulin G (IgG) scan

Anatomical and functional radioisotope imaging techniques are equally valuable in assessing patients with suspected mycotic aneurysms. Anatomical definition of the infectious process demonstrates the extent of infection, allows anticipation of technical difficulties, identifies safe locations for vascular clamp placement, and minimizes the likelihood of vascular injury or organ ischemia secondary to unsuspected anatomical anomalies or concomitant arterial occlusive disease. A caveat in patients with gastrointestinal hemorrhage associated with large abdominal aortic aneurysms is that a negative diagnostic imaging study does not exclude infection and the presence of a primary aortoenteric fistula.

ULTRASONOGRAPHY

Ultrasound scans can accurately depict aneurysms and complications of rupture, thrombosis, and arteriovenous fistula. Color Doppler flow imaging is particularly useful in evaluating pulsatile masses to differentiate between fluid collection or hematoma and false aneurysm formation. Diagnostic accuracy is dependent on the skill of the examiner, but the widespread availability of duplex scanners, coupled with the ability to perform bedside examinations of critically ill patients, make ultrasonography a useful initial diagnostic technique to verify vessel patency and size and to assess pulsatile masses adjacent to peripheral vessels, especially in the groin and limbs. Concomitant imaging of the venous system can be performed to verify patency and suitable-sized saphenous, internal jugular, and femoral veins for use as autologous grafts.

COMPUTED TOMOGRAPHY

Contrast-enhanced CT scanning is the preferred imaging technique in patients with suspected infection involving the aorta, or visceral or peripheral arteries. Diagnostic criteria of infection include well-

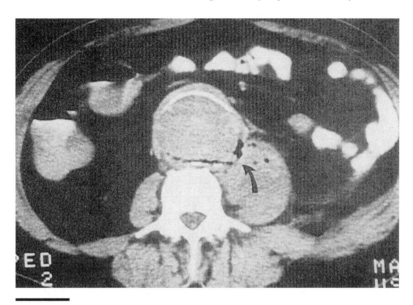

FIGURE 2.

Computed tomography scan of infected arotic aneurysm with gas *(arrow)* present within the aorta and adjacent soft tissue. Infected, confined aneurysmal rupture was found at surgery.

localized vessel dilatation with paucity of calcification, abnormal collections of fluid or air around the vessel wall, or an encasing mass that contains air, adjacent vertebral osteomyelitis, or juxta-aortic retroperitoneal abscess.[10] Computed tomographic-guided needle aspiration perivascular fluid collections is useful in identifying the infecting pathogen. Computed tomography scans are superior to ultrasound in the assessment of aneurysm wall integrity and the detection of inflammation or infection involving the aneurysm sac (Fig 2). Scanning can be performed with sufficient speed to be useful in evaluating symptomatic but hemodynamically stable patients with suspected rupture, or primary aortoduodenal fistula. Many hemorrhagic, embolic, and ischemic complications associated with operative management can be avoided with preliminary CT imaging. Arterial segments not involved in the inflammatory process can be accurately located and should be used as initial sites for dissection, vascular control, and placement of occluding clamps.

MAGNETIC RESONANCE IMAGING

MRI is a vascular imaging technique that affords anatomical delineation in multiple planes and provides information about tissue characterization (e.g., presence of fluid, inflammation). These features result in improved resolution between tissue and fluid interfaces compared to that with CT. Patients with suspected infection of the aorta can undergo scanning in transverse, sagittal, and coronal planes (Fig 3). Multiplanar reconstruction of vascular anatomy permits evaluation of complex aortic aneurysms. Anatomical information available includes lumen dimensions, rate of blood flow, quality of the aortic wall, cephalad and caudal extension, and involvement of branch vessels and neighboring structures. MRI has been demonstrated to be superior to CT in depicting the presence and extent of infection involving aortic grafts.[13] The ability to perform MR angiography with the scan data supports more widespread use of this modality for initial patient evaluation.

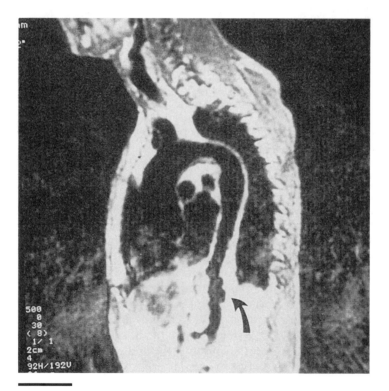

FIGURE 3.

Magnetic resonance image of thoracic and suprarenal aorta in a patient with tuberculous aortitis. Saccular dilatation of aorta was demonstrated in the sagittal view *(arrow)*.

ANGIOGRAPHY

Biplanar angiography should be performed on all patients with confirmed or suspected arterial infections. Angiograms can depict pseudoaneurysms, help assess patency of involved vessels or grafts, and help evaluate the status of proximal and distal vessels. A saccular or lobulated aneurysm of the aorta with otherwise normal vasculature is pathognomonic of a mycotic aneurysm (Fig 4). The diagnosis of intracranial or visceral mycotic aneurysms can only be made reliably with angiography. In most patients with arterial or vascular graft infections, angiography is used to plan surgical therapy and answer specific questions posed by results of clinical examination, or CT and MR imaging. If the facilities are available, intraarterial digital subtraction arteriography is the preferred initial angiographic technique.

FUNCTIONAL IMAGING TECHNIQUES

Radionuclide scans using ^{99m}Tc-labeled leukocytes, ^{111}In-labeled leukocytes, or polyclonal human IgG show accumulation at sites of infection.[11] False-positive accumulation of activity can occur in hematomas, pseudoaneurysms, tumors, and other sites of inflammation. False-negative results are unusual, but normal results have been reported in cases with primary aortoduodenal fistula and mycotic aneurysms with negative culture results. IgG scans are preferred over leukocyte scans because of ease of preparation, lack of staff exposure to patient blood, absence of concomitant erythrocyte and platelet imaging, and longer shelf life. Functional imaging studies can be used with MRI and CT imaging to accurately delineate the extent of infection. The accuracy of radioisotope scans in confirming the diagnosis of an infected aneurysm has not been evaluated.

MICROBIOLOGIC TESTING

Recovery of microorganisms from sites of suspected vascular infection is necessary to confirm the diagnosis and select antibiotic therapy. Appropriate microbiologic culture technique is important for the reliable recovery of aerobic and anaerobic bacteria, or fungi. Gram stain of tissue or perigraft fluid showing no organisms is not sufficient to exclude the presence of infection. Low numbers and virulence of infecting microorganisms, concomitant antibiotic administration, absence of tissue invasion, and activation of host defenses contribute to the sampling error or routine culture techniques. Use of tryptic soy broth media and mechanical (tissue grinding) explanted tissue reliably increase the recovery of micro-

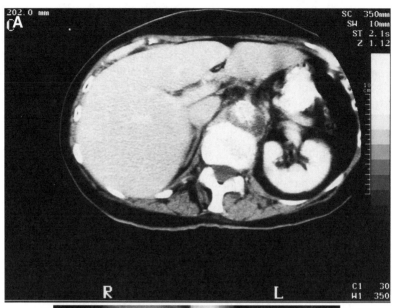

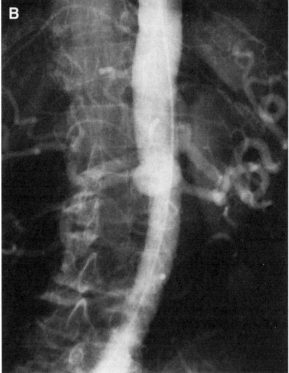

FIGURE 4.
Computed tomography scan **(A)** and aortogram **(B)** or a mycotic aneurysm
involving the visceral abdominal aorta in a patient with *S. aureus* septicemia.

organisms.[9] Culture tubes containing tissue specimens should be maintained for 5–7 days to exclude growth of coagulase-negative staphylococci.

MANAGEMENT STRATEGIES

Mycotic aneurysms are uniformly fatal if not treated with aggressive surgical and antibiotic therapy. The spectrum of vascular infection requires surgeons to individualize therapy based on the clinical presentation of the patient, anatomical location, and microbiologic characteristics of the infectious process (Fig 5).[2, 7, 9, 14–22] Early diagnosis permits en bloc excision of the aneurysm and periarterial infection, and allows a one-stage procedure with in situ replacement or ex-situ bypass. Delayed diagnosis with extensive perianeurysmal sepsis mandates excision and ligation often with a persistent risk of infection and arterial stump blow-out. When the thoracic or visceral abdominal aorta is involved, in situ reconstruction is the only feasible treatment coupled with prolonged (12 week) parenteral culture-specific antibiotic administration followed by lifetime suppressive antibiotic therapy. For infected aneurysms in the infrarenal aorta or peripheral arteries, excision, local debridement, and extraanatomic bypass is preferred, although in selected patients in situ reconstruction using autologous vein or a rifampin-bonded Dacron vascular prosthesis are therapeutic options. The quantity and virulence of pathogens, adequacy of local and systemic host defense mechanisms, and extent of the infectious process are critical factors that influence outcome. Residual arterial infection is the major cause of morbidity and mortality and the rea-

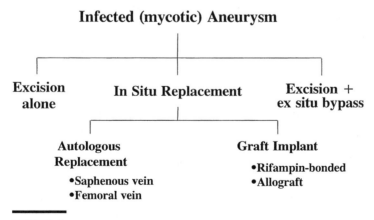

FIGURE 5.
Treatment options for mycotic aneurysms.

TABLE 2.

Antibiotic Therapy of Mycotic Aneurysms

	Antibiotic Administration	
Microorganism Isolated	**Perioperative (Parenteral)**	**Lifelong (Oral)**
None	Vancomycin, gentamicin	None
Staphylococcus/ streptococcus	Vancomycin, ampicillin/sulbactum	None
Gram-negative, polymicrobial	Culture-specific antibiotics	Culture-specific
Salmonella sp.	Ciprofloxin/Amoxicillin	Amoxacillin
Candida, fungi	Amphotericin B	Fluconazole

son local treatment methods and in situ grafting procedures often fail. Fichelle et al.[22] reported septic complication rates as high as 22% following in situ reconstruction. In general, local control of infection is more successful when there is absence of gross purulence, negative culture results, or *S. epidermidis* or fungi are recovered. Infections caused by gram-negative organisms, especially *Salmonella* sp and *Pseudomonas aeruginosa,* are associated with a high incidence (over 50%) of rupture, morbidity, and operative mortality.

Eradication of the infectious process and maintenance of adequate distal circulation are the two important principles of management. Systemic antibiotics bactericidal to bacteria recovered from blood or wound culture specimens, aspirated fluid, or expected pathogens should be administered (Table 2). Patients must be physiologically and psychologically prepared for surgery. Surgical control of infection is a priority when sepsis is present, because antibiotic administration alone is insufficient. In cases of ruptured aneurysms or primary aortoenteric fistula, operation should be undertaken immediately. The infected artery, aneurysm, or vascular graft must be totally excised and arterial reconstruction, if necessary, meticulously performed as either a staged or simultaneous procedure. Wide debridement of infected tissues, including the artery adjacent to the infectious process, antibiotic irrigation and placement of drains, reconstruction of vital arteries through uninfected tissue planes, and prolonged postoperative antibiotic administration are established surgical tenets. If a vascular infection can be excised without limb or organ loss, this treatment option is always preferred. In situ graft replacement (autologous vein, arterial homograft, antibiotic-impregnated prosthesis) is best suited for treatment of less virulent staphylococcal infections without extensive perivascular suppuration (Fig 6).

INFECTED AORTIC ANEURYSMS

For unruptured, infrarenal aortic infections, preliminary axillobifemoral bypass is the preferred initial procedure in hemodynamically stable patients when the diagnosis has been established.[12, 16] This approach eliminates lower limb ischemia and the necessity to administer heparin during excision of the aortic aneurysm or graft and closure of the aortic stump. The aorta should be debrided to normal-appearing tissue and closed using monofilament sutures. A pedicle of omentum is carefully positioned around the aortic stump and bed of excised aorta. Closed suction drains are left in the retroperitoneum and brought out of the flank opposite the axillofemoral graft.

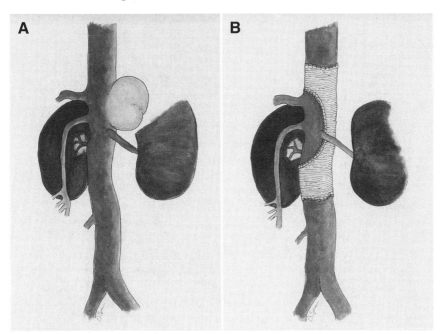

FIGURE 6.

Schematic drawing of *S. aureus* mycotic aneurysm involving visceral segment of the abdominal aorta **(A)**, and following in situ interposition grafting with a rifampin-bonded Dacron gelatin-impregnated graft spatulated onto the origins of the visceral/renal arteries.

When an infected aneurysm is complicated by contained rupture involving the visceral (suprarenal) aortic segment, a thoracoabdominal incision for a retroperitoneal approach to the aorta is preferred. This incision permits safe proximal aortic control, complete exposure of the involved aorta, and complex revascularization of vital organs, including autotransplantation of the left kidney to the iliac fossa. Vein grafts orginating from the iliac arteries that are perfused by an axillofemoral graft can be used to revascularize renal and mesenteric arteries.

Collected series over the past two decades strongly support the strategy of resection and remote bypass, but reoperation for extraanatomic graft complications (thrombosis, infection) and residual aortic infection manifest as aortic stump blowout remain major problems in the treatment of an infected aortic aneurysm. In situ prosthetic reconstruction has been used successfully in carefully selected patients with primary aortic infections, such as aortoduodenal fistula associated with large AAA.[7, 18, 19, 22] Relapsing infection is common with gram-negative infections, especially *Salmonella,* and presentation includes sepsis or rupture.

In the absence of gross purulence and sepsis, or when a low-grade infection is encountered (negative Gram's stain), in situ reconstruction using autologous reconstruction may be preferable to remote bypass using a prosthetic graft.[19–21, 24] This treatment option, which utilizes either arterial allograft or splicing segments of lower/upper extremity veins together, may not be feasible in all patients. The procedures are technically demanding but associated with perioperative morbidity similar to that of total graft excision and ex situ bypass. Benefits of in situ reconstruction include a reduced amputation rate, no aortic stump rupture, and avoidance of late complications (thrombosis, infection) of ex situ bypasses. In situ prosthetic graft replacement has been used successfully to treat both primary aortoenteric fistula. When infection involves the thoracic or suprarenal aorta and its branches, in situ graft replacement is the only practical approach. Use of a rifampin-impregnated Dacron graft is recommended when staphylococcal organisms are involved.[23, 24] A successful outcome has been reported in patients with gram-negative infection, including *Salmonella* after in situ prosthetic reconstruction, accompanied by thorough drainage and debridement, prolonged parenteral antibiotic (amoxicillin) therapy, and lifelong suppressive oral antibiotics.

FEMOROPOPLITEAL ARTERIAL SEGMENT

Collateral circulation is usually sufficient to maintain limb viability after excision and ligation of infected femoral artery aneurysms, particularly if limited to a single arterial segment—common, superficial, or deep. Autologous reconstruction using saphenous vein or an extra-anatomic (obturator canal, axillo-popliteal, iliac-superficial femoral) bypass can be used to reconstitute arterial flow to the lower limb when the entire femoral artery bifurcation must be excised (Fig 7). *S. aureus* and *Salmonella* sp. are the most common organisms isolated. The route of ex situ bypasses should completely avoid the septic area. Use of prosthetic grafts in drug addicts should be avoided, because continued drug use carries a high risk of graft infection. Recurrent infection following in situ autogenous vein grafting is disastrous, presenting as hemorrhage due to disruption of the vein graft wall.

CAROTID ARTERY

Ligation without reconstruction is safe when treating infected carotid or innominate artery aneurysms if carotid stump systolic pressure exceeds 70 mmHg. Temporary balloon occlusion in the angiography suite monitoring the patient's neurologic status can determine the safety of carotid occlusion. Direct autologous reconstruction using saphenous vein, or extracranial-to-intracranial bypass using saphenous vein or radial artey conduits may be required to maintain cerebral circulation in patients with poor hemispheric collaterals, vessels, depending on the extent and virulence of the carotid infection.

VISCERAL ARTERY

Treatment of mycotic aneurysms involving the visceral or renal arteries must be individualized and directed with angiography. The superior mesenteric artery is the most commonly involved visceral artery. Proximal and distal arterial control is obtained and the aneurysm excised if possible. Endoaneurysmorrhaphy with oversewing of the orifices of afferent and efferent vessels should be used when excision is not possible and for treatment of saccular aneurysms without purulence. This technique produces less damage to the collateral blood supply. Aneurysm excision and ligation of superior mesenteric, hepatic, celiac, and splenic arteries is the preferred procedure. Mesenteric revascularization is necessary if arterial insufficiency is produced after ligation. The preferred technique is use of saphenous vein graft originating from the

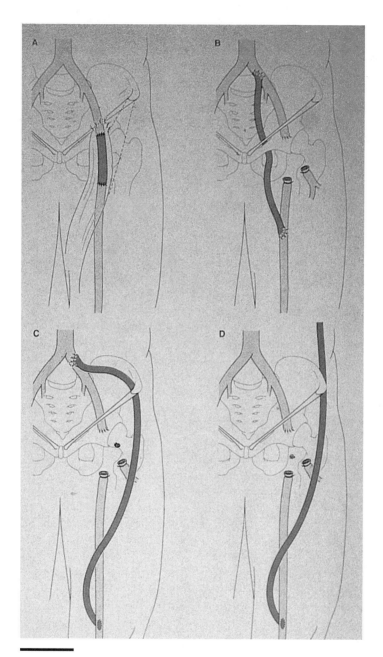

FIGURE 7.

Methods of femoral artery reconstruction after excision and ligation of femoral mycotic aneurysm. **A,** interposition vein autograft with sartorius muscle flap coverage. **B,** obturator bypass. **C,** lateral femoral bypass. **D,** unilateral axillofemoral bypass. (Courtesy of Reddy DJ, Smith RF, Elliott JP Jr, et al: Infected femoral artery false aneurysms in drug addicts: Evolution of selective vascular reconstruction. *J Vasc Surg* 3:718, 1986.)

TABLE 3.
Outcome of Treated Mycotic Aneurysms

| Study | Location (No.) | | Prevalent Pathogens | Surgical Treatment | Survivors |
	Aorta	Peripheral			
Jarrett et al, 1975[12]	12	—	*Staphylococcus* sp., *Salmonella* sp.	Excision + ex situ bypass	7 (59%)
Reddy et al, 1986[14]	—	54	*S. aureus*	Excision alone or + ex situ bypass	54 (100%)
Chan et al, 1989[2]	22	—	*S. aureus Salmonella* sp.	In situ repair	19 (86%)
Oz et al, 1989[15]	21	—	*Salmonella, Staphylococcus* sp.	Excision + in situ repair	
	7	—	*Streptococcus, S. aureus, Salmonella* sp.	Excision + in situ repair,	7 (100%)
Fichelle et al, 1993[22]	25	—	*Streptococcus* sp., *Salmonella* sp.	In situ repair (21) ex situ bypass (4)	21 (84%)
Hollier et al, 1993[13]	6	—	*S. aureus, Salmonella* sp.	Excision + in situ repair	5 (83%)
Vogt et al, 1996[25]	9	—	*S. aureus*	Excision + homograft replacement	9 (100%)

supraceliac aorta. Renal artery reconstruction is required to maintain organ function without exception.

RESULTS AND LATE OUTCOME

Early diagnosis coupled with careful preoperative and postoperative evaluation to assess etiology and extent of infection are key elements for successful treatment and long-term survival. Results after both excision and extraanatomic bypass and in situ reconstruction have improved because of advances in surgical technique and prolonged antimicrobial therapy (Table 3). Long-term survival with freedom from infection can be expected in most patients (over 75%). The amputation rate is 5% to 10% after treatment of aortic infections and 11% to 17% after excision of femoral mycotic aneurysm in drug addicts, compared to 30% to 50% after excision of infected infrainguinal bypass grafts. If the infectious process can be eradicated with artery excision, in situ replacement using implantation techniques and antibiotic-impregnated graft material that minimizes bacterial colonization may emerge as the preferred treatment. Recurrent or persistent infection is highest with salmonella infections and thus excision and ex situ grafting is recommended if feasible. The challenge of infected aneurysms can be answered when surgeons acquire in-depth understanding of etiologic mechanisms and the microorganisms likely to be involved, and are convinced that an aggressive approach can cure the majority of patients.

REFERENCES

1. Osler W: The Gulstonian lectures on malignant endocarditis. *Br Med J* 1:467, 1885.
2. Chan FY, Crawford ES, Coselli JS, et al: In situ prosthetic graft replacement for mycotic aneurysm of the aorta. *Ann Thorac Surg* 47:193, 1989.
3. Farooki MA: Aneurysms in the United States and the United Kingdom. *Int Surg* 58:475, 1973.
4. Sommerville RI, Allen EV, Edwards JE: Bland and infected arteriosclerotic abdominal aortic aneurysms: A clinicopathologic study. *Medicine* 38:207, 1959.
5. Patel S, Johnston W: Classification and management of mycotic aneurysms. *Surg Gynecol Obstet* 144:691, 1977.
6. Wilson SE, VanWagenen P, Passaro E Jr: Arterial infection. *Curr Probl Surg* 15:1, 1978.
7. Johansen K, Devin J: Mycotic aortic aneurysms: A reappraisal. *Arch Surg* 118:583, 1983.
8. Dean RH, Meacham PW, Weaver FA, et al: Mycotic embolism and embolomycotic aneurysms. *Ann Surg* 204:300, 1986.

9. Brown SL, Busittil RW, Baker JD, et al: Bacteriologic and surgical determinants of survival in patients with mycotic aneurysms. *J Vasc Surg* 1:541, 1984.
10. Blair RH, Resnik MD, Polga JP: CT appearance of mycotic abdominal aortic aneurysms. *J Comput Assist Tomogr* 13:101, 1989.
11. Fiorani P, Speziale F, Rizzo L, et al: Detection of aortic graft infection with leukocytes labelled with technetium 99m hexametazime. *J Vasc Surg* 17:87, 1993.
12. Jarrett F, Darling RC, Mundth ED, et al: Experience with infected aneurysms of the abdominal aorta. *Arch Surg* 110:1281, 1975.
13. Hollier LH, Money SR, Creely B, et al: Direct replacement of mycotic thoracoabdominal aneurysms. *J Vasc Surg* 18:477–485, 1993.
14. Reddy DJ, Smith RF, Elliott JP Jr, et al: Infected femoral artery false aneurysms in drug addicts: Evolution of selective vascular reconstruction. *J Vasc Surg* 3:718, 1986.
15. Oz MC, Brener BJ, Buda JA, et al: A ten-year experience with bacterial aortitis. *J Vasc Surg* 10:439, 1989.
16. Taylor LM Jr, Deitz DM, McConnell DB, et al: Treatment of infected abdominal aneurysms by extraanatomic bypass, aneurysm excision, and drainage. *Am J Surg* 155:655, 1988.
17. Feldman AJ, Berguer R: Management of an infected aneurysm of the groin secondary to drug abuse. *Surg Gynecol Obstet* 157:519, 1983.
18. Johnson JR, Ledgerwood AM, Lucas CE: Mycotic aneurysm: New concepts in therapy. *Arch Surg* 118:577, 1983.
19. Clagett GP, Bowers BL, Lopez-Viego MA, et al: Creation of a neo-aortoiliac system from lower extremity deep and superficial veins. *Ann Surg* 218:239, 1993.
20. Kieffer E, Bahnini A, Koskas F, et al: In situ allograft replacement of infected aortic prosthetic grafts: Results in forty-three patients. *J Vasc Surg* 176:349, 1993.
21. Torsello G, Sandmann W, Gehrt A, et al: In situ replacement of infected vascular prostheses with rifampin-soaked vascular grafts: Early results. *J Vasc Surg* 17:768, 1993.
22. Fichelle JM, Tabet G, Cormier P, et al: Infected infrarenal aortic aneurysms: When is in situ reconstruction safe. *J Vasc Surg* 17:635–645, 1993.
23. Gahtan V, Esses GE, Bandyk DF, et al: Antistaphylococcal activity of rifampin-bonded gelatin-impregnated Dacron grafts. *J Surg Res* 58:105–110, 1995.
24. Gupta AK, Bandyk DF, Johnson BL: In situ repair of mycotic abdominal aortic aneurysms with rifampin-bonded gelatin-impregnated Dacron grafts: A preliminary case report. *J Vasc Surg* 24:472–476, 1996.
25. Vogt PR, von Segesser LK, Goffin Y, et al: Eradication of aortic infections with the use of cryopreserved arterial homografts. *Ann Thorac Surg* 62:640–645, 1996.

PART VI

Minimally Invasive Techniques for the Lower Extremity

CHAPTER 11

Directional Atherectomy: Indications, Devices, Techniques, and Results

Stephen T. Kee, M.B., F.R.C.R.
Visiting Assistant Professor, Department of Cardiovascular and Interventional Radiology, Stanford University Hospital, Stanford, California

Charles P. Semba, M.D.
Department of Cardiovascular and Interventional Radiology, Stanford University Hospital, Stanford, California

Michael D. Dake, M.D.
Department of Cardiovascular and Interventional Radiology, Stanford University Hospital, Stanford, California

P ercutaneous atherectomy is the treatment of atherosclerotic arterial occlusive disease by catheter-based resection.[1] Although atherectomy devices use a variety of means of recanalization, the process is usually considered either extirpative or ablative.[2] Extirpative atherectomy involves shaving, cutting, or otherwise resecting atheromatous material from the patient and retrieving the resulting debris by suctioning the material through the device or by compacting it within a catheter collection chamber. Ablative atherectomy, on the other hand, removes the atheromatous plaque by using a high-speed rotational device to fragment or pulverize the atheroma into tiny particulate debris that is dispersed throughout the circulation. The devices discussed in this chapter on directional atherectomy are extirpative. Ablative devices are discussed elsewhere.

Atherectomy was developed to address some of the limitations associated with percutaneous balloon angioplasty, most notably restenosis.[3] After the initial experience was reported, it was considered a useful adjunct or alternative to balloon angioplasty. A num-

Advances in Vascular Surgery®, vol. 5
©1997, Mosby–Year Book, Inc.

ber of theoretical advantages of atherectomy over angioplasty were proposed:

1. Extension of endovascular treatment to lesions deemed relatively unsuitable for angioplasty (complete occlusion, eccentric lesions, fibrotic disease associated with dialysis access stenosis_ or bypass graft anastomotic disease).
2. Reduction in the restenosis rate as a result of removal, as opposed to compression, of the obstructing atheroma.
3. Lower frequency of intimal dissection without the necessity of plaque fracture.[3]

A wide variety of different endovascular systems have been developed for percutaneous atherectomy. The most widely used and reported system is the Simpson Peripheral AtheroCath (SPA), which is a prime example of an extirpative atherectomy device.[4] This device is the embodiment of the concept of percutaneous directional atherectomy because it allows image-guided, catheter-based resection directed at the precise areas of atheromatous narrowing rather than circumferential resection of the vessel wall.

This chapter will describe the basic design and mechanism of operation of currently available directional atherectomy devices, highlight the indications for their use, and present the long-term outcome of lesions treated by this technique.

SIMPSON PERIPHERAL ATHEROCATH

The most commonly used and evaluated atherectomy catheter is the SPA.[4] The device may be used as either a fixed-tip instrument (AtheroCath) or an over-the-wire catheter (AtheroTrac). It consists of a rotational cutter in a windowed housing with a positioning balloon mounted distally opposite the cutting window.

INDICATIONS FOR USE

The optimal lesion for the SPA is a focal eccentric stenosis in which the atheroma can be resected without affecting the relatively uninvolved portion of the vessel wall.[3] Concentric lesions and occluded vessels, although less ideal for this treatment, have been successfully recanalized.[5] The SPA can also be used to treat recurrent disease after angioplasty,[6] dialysis fistula stenosis,[7, 8] blue toe syndrome,[9] bypass graft stenosis,[10] and obstructing intimal flaps.[11] We have also used it to perform intraluminal vascular biopsies in cases in which the cause of obstruction is not known.[12, 13] In this regard, the most common clinical application in our experience is the di-

TABLE 1.
Working Diameters of Different-Sized
Atherectomy Catheters

French Size	Inflated Balloon Diameter, mm	Working Diameter, mm
7	3	5.3
7	4	6.3
8	3	5.7
8	5	7.7
9	3	6.0
9	5	8.0
10	4	7.3
10	6	9.3
11	4	7.7
11	6	9.7

agnosis of superior vena cava obstruction, particularly when an underlying malignancy is suspected.

The peripheral SPA device comes in a variety of French sizes, from 7F to 11F. The diameter of the positioning balloon varies with the size of the catheter and allows for a larger lumen to be treated than might be treated with the catheter alone (Table 1). The lesion to be treated must be in a segment of vessel that is accessible to the device. The system is fairly rigid; therefore, it is difficult to use via a contralateral iliac artery approach. A retrograde approach is used for iliac lesions, and an antegrade approach is used for femoral lesions.

TECHNIQUE

Because the majority of lesions to be treated are in the femoral or popliteal vessels, antegrade puncture of the ipsilateral common femoral artery is necessary. The rigid design of the device necessitates that vessel puncture be as horizontal as possible, which can prove extremely difficult in obese individuals. An appropriately sized sheath is inserted and the device advanced under fluoroscopic guidance to the abnormal region. The normal vessel caliber adjacent to the area of stenosis or occlusion should be determined in order to correctly select the size of the device. Sizing the device for the vessel concerned is critical inasmuch as undersizing results in excessive residual stenosis.[4] The AtheroCath is gently pushed through the vessel while the AtheroTrac can be advanced over a previously placed guidewire. Because the devices require relatively large introducer sheaths, IV heparin (5,000 units) is typically administered. To minimize arterial spasm, intra-arterial vasodilators such as nitroglycerin (100 to 200 mg) frequently are used.

The catheter has separate ports for flushing and balloon inflation (Fig 1). An inflator with a pressure gauge is used to inflate the balloon to 2 atm (218,000 Pa), and a separate motor drive is used to rotate the cutting blade at 2,000 rpm. An advancement control

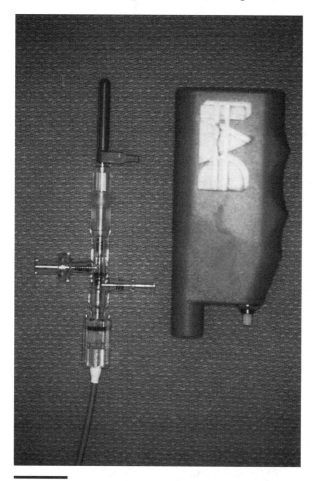

FIGURE 1.

The proximal end of the catheter shows the two ports, one for flushing and one for balloon inflation. Also shown is the disposable motor drive unit.

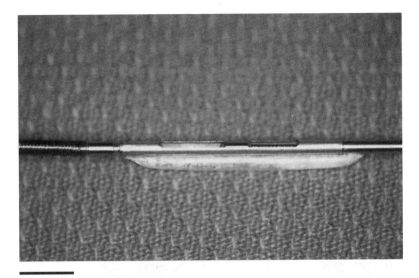

FIGURE 2.

The cutting end of the atherectomy catheter is shown with the rotating cutter partially advanced and the positioning balloon inflated.

lever is used to drive the cutting blade forward and backward.

Once the device is optimally positioned, the positioning balloon is inflated to 2 atm (218,000 Pa) to compress the cutting housing against the target atheroma. The handheld motor drive unit attached to the catheter is actuated. The rotating cutter is then advanced under continuous fluoroscopic guidance to shave the protruding plaque off the vessel (Fig 2). The atheromatous material is compressed into a collection chamber at the distal end of the device, where it remains until the device is removed.

When one surface of the vessel wall has been treated, the balloon is deflated and, if appropriate, the device rotated 30 to 40 degrees and the procedure repeated as necessary throughout the involved surface of the artery. When the collection chamber is full, there is a tactile sensation of resistance to complete advancement of the cutter. This is fluoroscopically apparent as the blade no longer advances into the collection chamber, which is packed full of debris. The device is then withdrawn to empty the collection chamber and perform an angiographic evaluation (Figs 3 to 6).

The windowed design helps prevent perforation when the device is being introduced because the cutting blade remains advanced within the housing and does not directly come in contact with the wall of the vessel until the lesion is crossed.

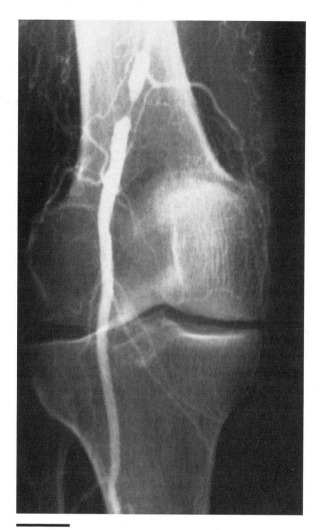

FIGURE 3.

Right leg arteriogram showing high-grade stenosis of the popliteal artery.

The fixed-tip device is useful for straight stenotic lesions, and the over-the-wire device is better for negotiating long, tortuous lesions. The over-the-wire mechanism is also more ideal when using the SPA to treat postangioplasty dissection.[14]

RESULTS

Initial technical success rates (less than 50% residual diameter stenosis after treatment) for this device range from 85% for the Athero-

Text continues on page 184

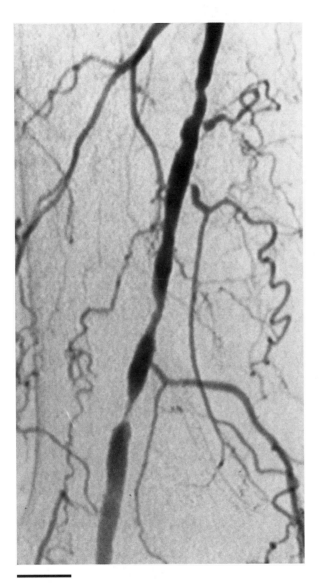

FIGURE 4.

Digital subtraction arteriogram of the right popliteal artery demonstrating the previously identified lesion and more proximal multifocal disease.

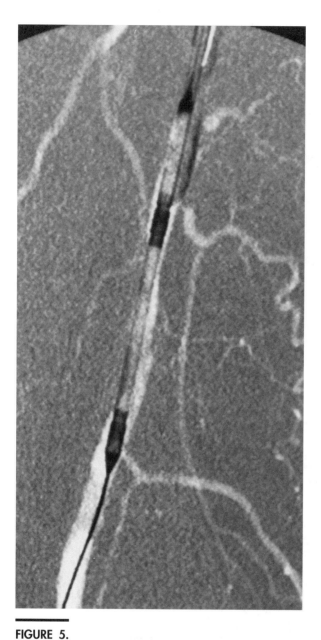

FIGURE 5.

Road map image of the popliteal artery with a 7F AtheroTrac device in place. The maximum diameter that can be achieved with this atherectomy catheter is 6.3 mm.

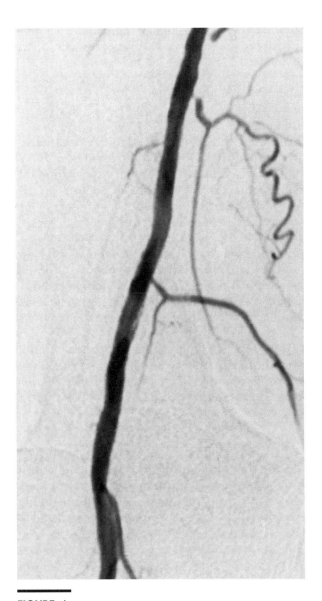

FIGURE 6.
Postatherectomy arteriogram showing a markedly improved popliteal artery lumen.

Cath to 100% for the over-the-wire AtheroTrac device.[1, 4, 5, 15–19] However, long-term clinical success has been somewhat disappointing, with a restenosis rate higher than that documented for percutaneous balloon angioplasty. For directional atherectomy, 2-year patency rates of 37% to 86% have been reported.[19–23] The major predictive factor for the development of restenosis is a persistent luminal stenosis of greater than 30% of the vessel diameter after atherectomy.[4] The optimal end point is stenosis less than 20% of the vessel diameter.[5]

In general, although the results of percutaneous atherectomy in various recent studies differ greatly, the overall results using the SPA device after 12 to 24 months' follow-up appear similar to those of conventional percutaneous transluminal angioplasty (PTA). In certain specific situations, the device appears to offer some benefit in treating eccentric, calcified lesions before angioplasty or stenting.

The SPA has been successfully used to treat stenoses involving the efferent venous outflow of arteriovenous fistulas. Many of the fibrotic stenoses encountered in the venous outflow tract of these fistulas behave in a similar fashion to calcified arterial lesions and are extremely resistant to balloon angioplasty. Directional atherectomy can be successfully used to resect the area of stenosis and preserve the fistula for further use.[7, 8]

The recent development and clinical adoption of endovascular stents have resulted in the abandonment of atherectomy for many formerly proposed indications, including the treatment of obstructing intimal flaps secondary to iatrogenic dissection.

COMPLICATIONS

The SPA device is associated with a low complication rate (3% to 7%).[4, 5, 16, 19, 24] A common complication is hematoma at the site of device introduction. In one series, dissection of the vessel wall was reported in only 3 of 61 patients.[4] Although distal embolization has been reported, no cases have required emergency surgery for this problem.[4, 19]

SUMMARY

The initial success rates of directional atherectomy using the SPA are similar to that of PTA; however, clinical follow-up at 6 and 12 months is disappointing, with a restenosis rate of about 30%. Although atherectomy is a theoretically attractive mechanical method for removing vessel plaque, the resultant trauma to the arterial wall appears to cause the development of intimal hyperplasia and associated poor long-term results. For this reason, its use cannot be recommended as a primary treatment modality for peripheral arterial occlusive disease because of its increased expense when compared with PTA and lack of improved clinical success rates when compared with more standard methods of care such as PTA, stenting, or surgery. Its use does retain value for certain specific applications, including arteriovenous fistula stenosis, endovascular biopsy, and intimal flap resection.

REFERENCES

1. Newman GE, Miner DG, Sussman SK, et al: Peripheral artery atherectomy: Description of technique and report of initial results. *Radiology* 169:677–680, 1988.
2. McLean GK: Percutaneous peripheral atherectomy. *J Vasc Interv Radiol* 4:465–480, 1993.
3. Ahn S: Peripheral atherectomy. *Semin Vasc Surg* 2:143–154, 1989.
4. Simpson JB, Selmon MR, Robertson GC, et al: Transluminal atherectomy for occlusive peripheral vascular disease. *Am J Cardiol* 61:96G–101G, 1988.
5. Graor RA, Whitlow PL: Transluminal atherectomy for occlusive peripheral vascular disease. *J Am Coll Cardiol* 15:1551–1558, 1990.
6. Korogi Y, Hirai T, Sakamoto Y, et al: Intravascular ultrasound imaging of peripheral arteries as an adjunct to atherectomy: Preliminary experience. *Br J Radiol* 68:110–115, 1995.
7. Zemel G, Katzen BT, Dake MD, et al: Directional atherectomy in the treatment of stenotic dialysis access fistulas. *J Vasc Interv Radiol* 1:35–38, 1990.
8. Gray RJ, Dolmatch BL, Buick MK: Directional atherectomy treatment for hemodialysis access: Early results. *J Vasc Interv Radiol* 3:497–503, 1992.
9. Dolmatch BL, Rholl KS, Moskowitz LB, et al: Blue toe syndrome: Treatment with percutaneous atherectomy. *Radiology* 173:799–804, 1989.
10. Vorwerk D, Guenther RW: Removal of intimal hyperplasia in vascular endoprostheses by atherectomy and balloon dilatation. *AJR Am J Roentgenol* 154:617–619, 1990.
11. Maynar M, Reyes R, Cabrera V, et al: Percutaneous atherectomy as an alternative for postangioplasty obstructive intimal flaps. *Radiology* 170:1029–1031, 1989.
12. Castaneda F, Moradian G, Hunter D, et al: Percutaneous intravascular biopsy using a Simpson atherectomy catheter: Technical note. *Cardiovasc Intervent Radiol* 12:342–343, 1990.
13. Dake M, Zemel G, Dolmatch B, et al: The cause of superior vena cava syndrome: Diagnosis with percutaneous atherectomy. *Radiology* 174:957–959, 1990.

14. Maynar M, Reyes R, Cabrera V, et al: Use of safety wire in atherectomy procedure for recanalization of complete arterial occlusions. *Semin Intervent Radiol* 5:256–261, 1988.
15. Belli AM, Cumberland DC: Percutaneous atherectomy—early experience in Sheffield. *Clin Radiol* 40:122–126, 1989.
16. Hofling B, Polnitz AV, Backa D, et al: Percutaneous removal of atheromatous plaques in peripheral arteries. *Lancet* 1:384–386, 1988.
17. Maynar M, Reyes R, Cabrera V, et al: Percutaneous atherectomy with the Simpson atherectomy device in the management of arterial stenosis. *Semin Intervent Radiol* 5:246–253, 1988.
18. Schwarten DE, Katzen BT, Simpson JB, et al: Simpson catheter for percutaneous transluminal removal of atheroma. *AJR Am J Roentgenol* 150:799–801, 1988.
19. von Polnitz A, Nerlich A, Berger H, et al: Percutaneous peripheral atherectomy: Angiographic and clinical follow-up of 60 patients [see comments]. *J Am Coll Cardiol* 15:682–688, 1990.
20. Dorros G, Iyer S, Lewin R, et al: Angiographic follow-up and clinical outcome of 126 patients after percutaneous directional atherectomy (Simpson AtheroCath) for occlusive peripheral vascular disease. *Cathet Cardiovasc Diagn* 22:79–84, 1991.
21. Graor R, Whitlow P: Directional atherectomy for peripheral vascular disease: Two year patency and factors influencing patency. *J Am Coll Cardiol* 17:106A, 1991.
22. Katzen B, Becker G, Benenati J, et al: Long-term follow-up of directional atherectomy in the femoral and popliteal arteries. *J Vasc Interv Radiol* 3:38, 1992.
23. Kim D, Gianturco LE, Porter DH, et al: Peripheral directional atherectomy: 4-year experience. *Radiology* 183:773–778, 1992.
24. Dorros G, Lewin RF, Sachdev N, et al: Percutaneous atherectomy of occlusive peripheral vascular disease: Stenoses and/or occlusions. *Cathet Cardiovasc Diagn* 18:1–6, 1989.

PART VII

Renal Artery Disease

CHAPTER 12

The Natural History of Renal Artery Disease

R. Eugene Zierler, M.D.

Professor of Surgery, Department of Surgery, Division of Vascular Surgery, University of Washington School of Medicine, Seattle, Washington

The relationship between renal artery stenosis and elevated blood pressure was first reported by Goldblatt et al.[1] in 1934, and renovascular disease continues to be the most common cause of secondary hypertension. It has been estimated that renovascular hypertension is present in 1% to 6% of unselected hypertensive patients.[2] In a study of 395 patients undergoing arteriography, renal artery stenosis of greater than 50% was found in 38% of the patients with abdominal aortic aneurysms, 33% of the patients with aortoiliac occlusive disease, and 39% of the patients with lower extremity arterial occlusive disease.[3] Atherosclerosis is the most common cause of renovascular disease in patients over the age of 50 years, and fibromuscular dysplasia is responsible for the majority of renal artery lesions in patients under the age of 40 years.

Many patients with renovascular hypertension can be treated effectively with antihypertensive drugs as long as their renal function remains stable. Whereas patients with fibromuscular dysplasia often derive long-term benefit from percutaneous transluminal angioplasty, patients with atherosclerotic renal artery stenosis are more prone to the development of recurrent stenotic lesions after angioplasty, even when intraluminal stents are used.[4, 5] Surgical bypass or endarterectomy of a renal artery lesion is usually reserved for patients resistant to antihypertensive drug therapy. Although the morbidity and mortality of renal artery surgery is extremely low in patients with nonatherosclerotic disease, the operative and late mortality among patients undergoing surgery for atherosclerotic renal artery lesions is significantly higher.[6, 7] Therefore, the decision to proceed with direct renal revascularization should be based on the risks of treatment, the expected outcome, and the known course of the disease without treatment.

Even when drug therapy is successful in controlling hypertension, an additional consequence of renal artery stenosis may be "ischemic nephropathy" leading to progressive renal insufficiency.[8, 9] Renal artery occlusive disease is estimated to be the primary cause of end-stage renal failure in 5% to 15% of the patients older than 50 years of age who begin dialysis each year.[10, 11] Clinical experience indicates that renal revascularization permitting withdrawal from or avoidance of dialysis results in improved long-term survival.[12, 13]

NATURAL HISTORY STUDIES

Natural history studies are designed to provide detailed information on the clinical outcome of a disease without treatment. The characteristic feature of a natural history study is serial follow-up of patients to document both the initial severity of their disease and any subsequent changes that occur over time. Such studies are helpful in the evaluation of therapeutic interventions because they make it possible to determine whether a particular treatment results in a better clinical outcome than no treatment at all. The value of renal revascularization in patients with severe renal artery disease and established renovascular hypertension or ischemic renal failure is generally accepted. However, the role of intervention for renal artery stenosis that is not associated with uncontrollable hypertension or decreased renal function remains uncertain. Thus, the ultimate goal of natural history studies on renal artery disease is to provide a rationale for managing patients with asymptomatic or minimally symptomatic renal artery stenosis.

Because natural history studies require frequent evaluations of relatively large numbers of patients, the risks and costs of the testing methods used are of critical importance. Clinicians have been reluctant to use arteriography as a routine screening test for renal artery stenosis in patients with suspected renovascular hypertension or renal failure because of its high cost, the risk of arterial puncture, and the nephrotoxicity of radiographic contrast material. Noninvasive testing methods are ideally suited for screening and follow-up examinations in natural history studies. The critical requirement of a noninvasive method is that it be sufficiently accurate to provide meaningful clinical data.

A variety of indirect and direct noninvasive diagnostic tests are available for assessing the extracranial carotid system, the peripheral arteries, and the peripheral veins.[14] However, there are no indirect techniques for evaluating the renal or mesenteric vessels, so it was not until the development of abdominal duplex scanning that renal artery disease could be reliably identified by noninvasive means.[15] This has made it possible to conduct definitive natural history studies on renal artery disease.

The technique of renal duplex scanning has been described in detail previously.[15–19] B-mode and color-flow images are used to locate the renal arteries, and the severity of disease is determined by inspection of pulsed Doppler spectral waveforms. As for duplex scanning in other areas of the arterial system, identification of stenotic lesions in the renal arteries is based on the presence of a localized high-velocity jet and poststenotic turbulence. Comparisons between duplex scanning and arteriography show overall accuracies in the range of 81% to 97% for the detection of significant renal artery disease.[17–19] The clinical applications of renal duplex scanning include screening of selected patients with hypertension, screening of selected patients with renal failure, intraoperative assessment, follow-up of renal revascularization, evaluation of renal transplants, and natural history studies.

RETROSPECTIVE STUDIES

Most of the published reports on the prevalence and natural history of renal artery disease are based on autopsy studies or selected patients undergoing arteriography. Holley et al. found moderate or severe renal artery stenosis at autopsy in 53% of 295 patients, including 49% of 256 normotensive patients and 77% of 39 patients with a history of hypertension.[20] Severe renal artery stenosis increased in frequency with age and was uncommon in patients younger than 50 years of age. Among 500 patients undergoing arteriography for a variety of vascular problems, Eyler et al. observed renal artery abnormalities in 219, or 44%.[21] Renal artery lesions were present in 32% of 304 normotensive patients and 62% of 196 patients with hypertension. Another arteriographic study reported by Brewster et al. documented renal artery stenoses in 22% of their patients with abdominal aortic aneurysms.[22]

Because they include only patients requiring multiple arteriograms, natural history studies based on serial arteriography may overestimate the true incidence of renal artery disease progression. In a review by Meaney et al. of 39 patients with atherosclerotic renal artery lesions who underwent serial arteriography at intervals ranging from 6 months to 10 years, an increase in stenosis severity was noted in 10 and renal artery thrombosis occurred in 4, for an overall progression rate of 36%.[23] A similar study by Wollenweber et al. monitored 30 patients for a mean period of 42 months and documented progression in 50% of the renal artery lesions.[24] Schreiber et al. monitored 85 patients with serial arteriography for a mean period of 52 months and showed progression of atherosclerotic renal artery stenosis in 37 patients, or 44%, including 14 patients in whom total renal artery occlusion developed.[25] The risk of progression to occlusion was particularly high for renal arteries with more than 75% stenosis on the initial arteriogram. In the latter two studies, deterioration in renal function and a decrease in renal size were both more common in patients showing progression of renal artery disease than in patients with stable renal artery lesions.

Tollefson and Ernst studied 48 patients with atherosclerotic renal artery stenosis who underwent serial arteriography for aortic disease but did not have repair of the renal artery lesions.[26] All patients had at least two arteriograms separated by an interval of 1 year or more, and the mean follow-up period was 7.3 years. Of the 79 renal artery lesions identified, progression of stenosis was seen in 42, or 53%. The overall rate of progression was 4.6% per year. Seven lesions (9%) progressed to total occlusion, and all 7 had stenoses averaging 80% before occlusion. No renal artery stenoses of less than 60% progressed directly to occlusion.

Although relatively few reports deal with the natural history of renal artery fibromuscular dysplasia, the available retrospective studies suggest that fibromuscular lesions are less likely to progress than atherosclerotic renal artery disease.[4, 23, 25] Meaney et al. observed worsening of renal artery fibromuscular dysplasia in 8 of 51 patients, for an overall progression rate of 16%.[23] Of the 66 patients monitored by Schreiber et al., progression of renal artery fibromuscular dysplasia occurred in 22, or 33%.[25] In contrast to atherosclerotic renal artery disease, progression to renal artery occlusion or renal insufficiency appears to be extremely rare in patients with fibromuscular dysplasia. Spontaneous regression of fibromuscular renal artery lesions with reversal of hypertension has also been described.[27]

Although the natural history studies just summarized provide some useful data, they are retrospective in design and used arteriography as the method for identifying patients with renal artery stenosis. Because indications for arteriography were required, the patients were highly selected and do not necessarily represent the general population of patients with renal artery disease.

PROSPECTIVE STUDIES

Successful application of duplex scanning for documenting the natural history of carotid artery disease suggested that the same approach could be used for the renal artery.[28] In a small prospective study, duplex scanning was used to monitor 27 patients with 35 renal artery stenoses involving 60% to 99% diameter reduction.[29] Of these, 19 lesions were observed without intervention for a mean of 13 months. Although all 19 stenotic renal arteries remained patent during the follow-up period, ipsilateral kidney length decreased by a mean of 1.0 cm. There was no significant change in length for kidneys with nonstenotic renal arteries. Sixteen renal artery stenoses were monitored in the same study after interventions. Six arteries in 5 patients were treated by percutaneous transluminal angioplasty, and surgical bypass was performed on 10 arteries in 7 patients. The angioplasty group was monitored for a mean of 6.5 months. Duplex scanning documented relief of renal artery stenosis in 2 patients whose hypertension improved after angioplasty and persistent stenosis in 3 patients whose hypertension did not improve. Follow-up of the surgical bypass group for a mean of 9 months showed 8 patent and 2 occluded grafts.

Based on the aforementioned preliminary experience, a prospective natural history study was initiated in the vascular research laboratory at the University of Washington. The study population consists of patients with atherosclerotic renal artery disease identified by duplex scanning who do not require immediate intervention. The severity of stenosis for each renal artery is classified into one of four categories according to the criteria in Table 1. These criteria are based on the maximum peak systolic velocity in the renal artery and the ratio of the peak systolic velocity in the renal artery to that in the adjacent abdominal aorta (renal-aortic ratio). The renal artery disease categories are normal, less than 60% di-

---

TABLE 1.

Criteria for Classification of Renal Artery Disease by Duplex Scanning

Renal Artery Diameter Reduction	Renal Artery PSV	RAR
Normal	<180 cm/sec	<3.5
<60%	≥180 cm/sec	<3.5
≥60%	</≥180 cm/sec	≥3.5
Occlusion (100%)	No signal	No signal

Abbreviations: PSV, peak systolic velocity; *RAR,* renal/aortic ratio (ratio of the peak systolic velocity in the renal artery to the peak systolic velocity in the adjacent abdominal aorta).

ameter reduction, 60% diameter reduction or greater, and occlusion. Eligible patients must have at least one abnormal renal artery with a peak systolic velocity of ≥ 180 cm/sec or a renal-aortic ratio of ≥ 3.5. Evaluations are performed at 6-month intervals for patients with at least one high-grade (60% or greater diameter reduction) renal artery stenosis and 12-month intervals for patients with less severe lesions.

At baseline and at each follow-up evaluation, a detailed medical questionnaire is completed and a renal duplex scan is performed. The renal duplex scan includes an assessment of both renal arteries, the abdominal aorta, the renal parenchyma, and measurement of kidney lengths. A carotid artery duplex scan and noninvasive evaluation of the lower extremity arterial circulation are also done to assess the prevalence and progression rate of atherosclerosis in other segments of the arterial circulation. Finally, a blood specimen is obtained for determination of serum blood urea nitrogen, creatinine, and lipid levels.

For the purposes of this study, disease progression in a renal artery is defined as an increase in stenosis severity on serial duplex examinations to 60% or greater diameter reduction or occlusion. Thus, renal arteries that are normal or have less than 60% stenosis at the baseline evaluation show disease progression if they are found to have either 60% or greater stenosis or occlusion during follow-up. Renal arteries with 60% or greater stenosis at baseline can only progress to occlusion. If a renal artery is occluded at the baseline evaluation, no further disease progression is possible. Because eligible patients may have only one abnormal renal artery and both renal arteries are monitored in the study protocol, follow-up data are available on some contralateral normal renal arteries.

Progression of Renal Artery Stenosis

A detailed report on the first 80 patients enrolled in the University of Washington study was published in 1994.[30] The patient group included 36 males and 44 females with a mean age of 66 years. Most of these patients were originally referred for renal artery screening because of hypertension or decreased renal function. At the baseline evaluation, 42% of the patients had coronary artery disease, 41% had lower extremity arterial disease, 38% had extracranial carotid artery disease, and 10% had diabetes mellitus. Based on a strict clinical threshold of 140/90 mm Hg, only 6% of the patients would be considered to have had adequate blood pressure control at the time of entry into the study. Of the 139 renal arteries eligible for follow-up, the baseline duplex scan was classified as normal in 36, less than 60% stenosis in 35, 60% or greater stenosis in 63, and occlusion in 5. The mean follow-up interval at the time of reporting was 12.7 months, with a maximum follow-up of 26 months. None of the 36 renal arteries that were normal at the baseline evaluation showed disease progression to either 60% or greater stenosis or occlusion. Seven of the 35 renal arteries with less than 60% stenosis at baseline progressed to 60% or greater stenosis during the follow-up period. The cumulative incidence of progression to 60% or greater stenosis was 23% at 12 months and 42% at 24 months. All 4 of the renal arteries that progressed to occlusion had 60% or greater stenosis at the baseline evaluation, for a cumulative incidence of progression from 60% or greater stenosis to occlusion of 5% at 12 months and 11% at 24 months.

An updated review of the renal artery disease progression data has recently been reported.[31] After exclusion of 4 women with possible fibromuscular dysplasia, the patient group includes 76 patients (36 males, 40 females) with a mean age of 67 years who have been monitored for a mean interval of 32 months (maximum, 55 months). The baseline status of the 132 patent renal arteries eligible for follow-up was normal in 36, less than 60% stenosis in 35, and 60% or greater stenosis in 61. The cumulative incidence of progression from normal to 60% or greater stenosis was 0% at 1 year, 0% at 2 years, and 8% at 3 years (Table 2). The cumulative incidence of progression from less than 60% to 60% or greater stenosis was 30% at 1 year, 44% at 2 years, and 48% at 3 years. For those arteries with 60% or greater stenosis, the cumulative incidence of progression to occlusion was 4% at 1 year, 4% at 2 years, and 7% at 3 years.

The categorical and continuous risk factors that were evaluated for predictive value relative to progression of renal artery stenosis are listed in Tables 3 and 4. The following risk factors showed trends toward an association with progression of renal artery stenosis: advanced age, elevated systolic blood pressure, pack-years of smoking, female sex, poorly controlled blood pressure (>140/90 mm Hg), and a history of carotid endarterectomy.

Changes in Kidney Length

One goal of the ongoing natural history study is to determine the changes in kidney length that occur in patients with atherosclerotic renal artery disease. To establish what should be considered

TABLE 2.

Cumulative Incidence of Renal Artery Disease Progression

	Follow-up Interval			
Baseline Renal Duplex	**0 mo**	**12 mo**	**24 mo**	**36 mo**
Normal				
Progression (0.95 CI)	0%	0%	0%	8% (0–19)
n	36	33	27	22
<60% stenosis				
Progression (0.95 CI)	0%	30% (15–45)	44% (25–63)	48% (28–68)
n	35	22	14	11
≥60% stenosis				
Progression (0.95 CI)	0%	4% (0–9)	4% (0–9)	7% (0–16)
n	61	43	31	20
All progressions				
Progression (0.95 CI)	0%	10% (5–15)	14% (7–21)	20% (12–28)
n	132	98	72	53

Abbreviations: CI, confidence interval; *n,* number of renal arteries at the beginning of the follow-up interval.

(Reprinted by permission of Elsevier Science Inc. from Zierler RE, Bergelin RO, Davidson RC, et al: A prospective study of disease progression in patients with renal artery stenosis, *AMERICAN JOURNAL OF HYPERTENSION,* 9:1055–1061. Copyright 1996 by American Journal of Hypertension, Inc.)

a significant change, the variability of duplex ultrasound kidney length measurements was determined.[32] Using normal subjects, a single examiner, and the same duplex scanner, the standard deviation of the difference between kidney length measurements was found to be 0.45 cm. Based on this figure, kidney length changes of more than 1 cm were considered to be significant in the natural history study. Early experience with serial duplex scanning indicated that the presence of severe ipsilateral renal artery stenosis is associated with a significant decrease in kidney length over time.[33]

Data on changes in kidney length are now available on 123 patients (55 males, 68 females) with a mean age 68 years who had been evaluated at 6-month intervals for an average of 31.3 months (maximum, 72 months). Of the 225 renal artery and kidney sides that were monitored, 34 (15%) were found to have greater than a 1-cm decrease in length. Among the remaining sides, 173 (77%) did not decrease in size, and 18 (8%) were already small (<8.5 cm

TABLE 3.

Association of Categorical Risk Factors
With Renal Artery Disease Progression

Baseline Risk Factor	Disease Progression, %	P Value
Sex		
Male (36)*	31	0.05
Female (40)	52	
Blood pressure control		
>140/90 (66)	47	0.13†
≤140/90 (8)	13	
Current/former smoker		
No (19)	42	1.00
Yes (57)	42	
Diabetes mellitus		
No (68)	40	0.27†
Yes (8)	62	
Myocardial infarction		
No (50)	40	0.61
Yes (26)	46	
Intermittent claudication		
No (69)	42	1.00†
Yes (7)	43	
Carotid endarterectomy		
No (68)	38	0.06†
Yes (8)	75	
High cholesterol		
No (45)	42	0.90
Yes (27)	41	

*Sample size in parentheses.
†P Value computed by the two-tailed Fisher's exact test.
(Reprinted by permission of Elsevier Science Inc. from Zierler RE, Bergelin RO, Davidson RC, et al: A prospective study of disease progression in patients with renal artery stenosis, *AMERICAN JOURNAL OF HYPERTENSION,* 9:1055–1061. Copyright 1996 by American Journal of Hypertension, Inc.)

TABLE 4.

Association of Continuous Risk Factors With Presence or Absence
of Renal Artery Disease Progression

Baseline Risk Factor	Disease Progression		*P* Value
	No, Mean ± SD	Yes, Mean ± SD	
Age	66 ± 9 (44)*	69 ± 8 (32)	0.08
Systolic blood pressure	164 ± 22 (43)	171 ± 20 (32)	0.15
Diastolic blood pressure	85 ± 7 (43)	85 ± 10 (32)	0.87
BUN	21 ± 10 (32)	26 ± 22 (26)	0.26[+]
Creatinine	1.3 ± 0.6 (32)	1.6 ± 1.6 (26)	0.39
Pack-years of smoking	27 ± 30 (39)	39 ± 37 (28)	0.14

*Sample size in parentheses.
[+]Distribution of BUN values is markedly skewed; the Mann-Whitney *P* value is 1.00.
Abbreviations: SD, standard deviation; *BUN,* blood urea nitrogen.
(Reprinted by permission of Elsevier Science Inc. from Zierler RE, Bergelin RO, Davidson
RC, et al: A prospective study of disease progression in patients with renal artery steno-
sis, *AMERICAN JOURNAL OF HYPERTENSION,* 9:1055–1061. Copyright 1996 by Ameri-
can Journal of Hypertension, Inc.)

in length) at the time of entry into the study. For kidneys with a
60% or greater renal artery stenosis at the baseline evaluation, 21%
showed greater than a 1-cm decrease in length during follow-up.
The corresponding figures for sides with less than 60% stenosis
and normal renal arteries at baseline were 12% and 6%, respectively. Among those sides that were initially less than 60% stenotic
or normal, a decrease greater than 1 cm in length was significantly
more common when renal artery disease progression was observed
during the follow-up period. There was a strong association
between 60% or greater renal artery stenosis, low renal parenchy-
mal blood flow velocities, and a significant decrease in kidney
length during follow-up. Other factors that appear to be associated
with renal atrophy include a low ankle-arm index, systolic hypertension, and diabetes. All 7 of the renal arteries that progressed to
occlusion during follow-up had 60% or greater stenosis, and the
mean kidney length before occlusion was 8.5 cm. This is in contrast to a mean kidney length of 9.5 cm for those kidneys that decreased in size while their arteries remained patent.

These data, although still preliminary, suggest that patients
with high-grade renal artery stenoses or progression of atherosclerotic renal artery disease are at risk for a significant decrease in

kidney length. This loss of renal mass may have important consequences for overall renal function. Features that could ultimately influence the decision to recommend renal revascularization in this setting include absolute kidney length, rate of kidney shrinkage, severity of renal artery stenosis, degree of renal insufficiency, and rate of decline in renal function. Based on the association between small kidneys and renal artery occlusion, the concept of a size threshold for intervention appears to have some validity. The natural history data suggest that maximum benefit should be obtained when a revascularized kidney is at least 8.5 to 9 cm in length. The presence of low blood flow velocities in the renal parenchyma is another duplex US parameter that may prove to be useful in predicting which kidneys are at highest risk for significant decreases in length.[34]

Prevalence of Carotid and Lower Extremity Atherosclerosis

Because atherosclerosis is a widespread systemic disease, patients with atherosclerotic renal artery stenosis would be expected to show atherosclerotic involvement in other segments of the arterial system. The prevalence of extracranial carotid and lower extremity arterial occlusive disease was evaluated in a subset of 60 patients (25 males, 35 females) in the renal artery natural history study.[35] Carotid disease was assessed by duplex scanning, and the severity of lower extremity involvement was assessed by the ankle-brachial index (ABI). Fifty-two patients had one or more renal artery stenoses of 60% or greater, and 8 patients had less severe renal artery lesions. For those patients with 60% or greater renal artery stenoses, 25 (46%) had 50% or greater stenosis of one or both internal carotid arteries, and 27 (54%) had lesser degrees of carotid disease. Among patients with less than 60% renal artery stenosis, only 2 (25%) had high-grade internal carotid artery stenoses whereas 6 (75%) had lesser degrees of carotid disease. For the lower extremities, an ABI of 0.95 or greater was considered normal and an ABI of less than 0.95 was used as an indicator of significant arterial occlusive disease. Of the patients with 60% or greater renal artery stenosis, 38 (73%) had an ABI less than 0.95 and 14 (27%) had a normal ABI. For the patients with less than 60% renal artery stenosis, 4 (50%) had a normal ABI and 4 (50%) had an ABI less than 0.95.

These data confirm the high prevalence of carotid and lower extremity arterial occlusive disease in patients with atherosclerotic renal artery stenosis. The prevalence of these lesions is especially high in patients with severe renal artery stenoses. Patients being evaluated and treated for renal artery disease need to be screened appropriately for arterial lesions in these other areas.

CONCLUSIONS

Retrospective studies on the natural history of renal artery stenosis suggest that disease progression occurs in 30% to 50% of patients monitored for mean periods of up to 7 years. In the ongoing University of Washington natural history study, progression of renal artery stenosis occurred at an average rate of 7% per year for all categories of baseline disease combined. Although progression of disease in renal arteries that were initially normal was rare, the cumulative incidence of progression from less than 60% to 60% or greater renal artery stenosis was 30% at 12 months, 44% at 24 months, and 48% at 36 months. The cumulative incidence of progression from 60% or greater stenosis to occlusion was 4% at 12 months, 4% at 24 months, and 7% at 36 months. It is also noteworthy that indications for renal artery intervention developed in 9% of the patients recruited for the study after entry into the follow-up protocol.

Although no definitive clinical recommendations can be made on the basis of the current natural history data, it is clear that progression of atherosclerotic renal artery stenosis is common, particularly from less than 60% to 60% or greater stenosis. A relatively low but consistent rate of progression from 60% or greater stenosis to renal artery occlusion has also been observed. The combination of severe renal artery stenosis and a small kidney appears to be associated with a higher risk of progression to renal artery occlusion. Patients with 60% or greater renal artery stenosis or progression of renal artery disease are at risk for significant decreases in kidney length. Although these findings suggest that early renal revascularization may be beneficial for selected patients with severe renal artery stenoses, the effect of such intervention on further disease progression, changes in kidney size, and clinical outcome remains to be established. Additional data from natural history studies should help refine the patient selection criteria and provide more specific guidelines for intervention.

REFERENCES

1. Goldblatt H, Lynch J, Hanzai RF, et al: Studies on experimental hypertension I. The production of persistent elevation of systolic blood pressure by means of renal ischemia. *J Exp Med* 59:347–379, 1934.

2. Simon N, Franklin SS, Bleifer KH, et al: Clinical characteristics of renovascular hypertension. *JAMA* 220:1209–1218, 1972.

3. Olin JW, Melia M, Young JR, et al: Prevalence of atherosclerotic renal artery stenosis in patients with atherosclerosis elsewhere. *Am J Med* 88:46N–51N, 1990.

4. Lüscher TF, Lie JT, Stanson AW, et al: Arterial fibromuscular dysplasia. *Mayo Clin Proc* 62:931–952, 1987.

5. Tullis MJ, Zierler RE, Glickerman DJ, et al: Results of percutaneous transluminal angioplasty for atherosclerotic renal artery stenosis: A follow-up study with duplex ultrasonography. *J Vasc Surg* 25:46–54, 1997.

6. Anderson CA, Hansen KJ, Benjamin ME, et al: Renal artery fibromuscular dysplasia: Results of current surgical therapy. *J Vasc Surg* 22:207–216, 1995.

7. Hansen KJ, Starr SM, Sands RE, et al: Contemporary surgical management of renovascular disease. *J Vasc Surg* 16:319–331, 1992.

8. Jacobson HR: Ischemic renal disease: An overlooked clinical entity. *Kidney Int* 34:729–743, 1988.

9. Dean RH, Tribble RW, Hansen KJ, et al: Evolution of renal insufficiency in ischemic nephropathy. *Ann Surg* 213:446–456, 1991.

10. Rimmer JM, Gennari J: Atherosclerotic renovascular disease and progressive renal failure. *Ann Intern Med* 118:712–719, 1993.

11. O'Neil EA, Hansen KJ, Canzanello VJ, et al: Prevalence of ischemic nephropathy in patients with renal insufficiency. *Ann Surg* 58:485–490, 1992.

12. Kaylor WM, Novick AC, Ziegelbaum M, et al: Reversal of end-stage renal failure with surgical revascularization in patients with atherosclerotic renal artery occlusion. *J Urol* 141:486–488, 1989.

13. Hansen KJ, Thomason RB, Craven TE, et al: Surgical management of dialysis-dependent ischemic nephropathy. *J Vasc Surg* 1:197–211, 1995.

14. Zierler RE: The role of the vascular laboratory in clinical decision-making. *Semin Roentgenol* 27:63–77, 1992.

15. Kohler TR, Zierler RE, Martin RL, et al: Noninvasive diagnosis of renal artery stenosis by ultrasonic duplex scanning. *J Vasc Surg* 4:450–456, 1986.

16. Taylor DC, Kettler MD, Moneta GL, et al: Duplex ultrasound in the diagnosis of renal artery stenosis—a prospective evaluation. *J Vasc Surg* 7:363–369, 1988.

17. Hoffmann U, Edwards JM, Carter S, et al: Role of duplex scanning for the detection of atherosclerotic renal artery disease. *Kidney Int* 39:1232–1239, 1991.

18. Hansen KJ, Tribble RW, Reavis S, et al: Renal duplex sonography: Evaluation of clinical utility. *J Vasc Surg* 12:227–236, 1990.

19. Olin JW, Piedmonte MR, Young JR, et al: The utility of duplex ultrasound scanning of the renal arteries for diagnosing significant renal artery stenosis. *Ann Intern Med* 122:833–838, 1995.

20. Holley KE, Hunt JC, Brown AL, et al: Renal artery stenosis—a clinical-pathologic study in normotensive and hypertensive patients. *Am J Med* 37:14–22, 1964.
21. Eyler WR, Clark MD, Garman JF, et al: Angiography of the renal areas including a comparative study of renal arterial stenoses in patients with and without hypertension. *Radiology* 78:879–891, 1962.
22. Brewster DC, Retana A, Waltman AC, et al: Angiography in the management of aneurysms of the abdominal aorta—its value and safety. *N Engl J Med* 292:822–825, 1975.
23. Meaney TF, Dustan HP, McCormack LJ: Natural history of renal arterial disease. *Radiology* 91:881–887, 1968.
24. Wollenweber J, Sheps SG, Davis GD: Clinical course of atherosclerotic renovascular disease. *Am J Cardiol* 21:60–71, 1968.
25. Schreiber MJ, Pohl MA, Novick AC: The natural history of atherosclerotic and fibrous renal artery disease. *Urol Clin North Am* 11:383–392, 1984.
26. Tollefson DF, Ernst CB: Natural history of atherosclerotic renal artery stenosis associated with aortic disease. *J Vasc Surg* 14:327–331, 1991.
27. Siegler RL, Miller FJ, Mineau DE, et al: Spontaneous reversal of hypertension caused by fibromuscular dysplasia. *J Pediatr* 100:83–85, 1982.
28. Roederer GO, Langlois YE, Jager KA, et al: The natural history of carotid arterial disease in asymptomatic patients with cervical bruits. *Stroke* 15:605–613, 1984.
29. Taylor DC, Moneta GL, Strandness DE Jr: Follow-up of renal artery stenosis by duplex ultrasound. *J Vasc Surg* 9:410–415, 1989.
30. Zierler RE, Bergelin RO, Isaacson JA, et al: Natural history of atherosclerotic renal artery stenosis: A prospective study with duplex ultrasonography. *J Vasc Surg* 19:250–258, 1994.
31. Zierler RE, Bergelin RO, Davidson RC, et al: A prospective study of disease progression in patients with atherosclerotic renal artery stenosis. *Am J Hypertens* 9:1055–1061, 1996.
32. Isaacson JA, Zierler RE, Bergelin RO, et al: A method for minimizing variability in kidney length measurements during renal artery duplex scanning. *J Vasc Technol* 18:23–27, 1994.
33. Guzman RP, Zierler RE, Isaacson JA, et al: Renal atrophy and arterial stenosis: A prospective study with duplex ultrasound. *Hypertension* 23:346–350, 1994.
34. Louie J, Isaacson JA, Zierler RE, et al: Hemodynamic parameters for diagnosis of advanced renal artery stenosis by duplex ultrasound. *J Vasc Technol* 18:61–66, 1994.
35. Louie J, Isaacson JA, Zierler RE, et al: Prevalence of carotid and lower extremity arterial disease in patients with renal artery stenosis. *Am J Hypertens* 7:436–439, 1994.

PART VIII

Issues in Basic Science

CHAPTER 13

Options for Anticoagulation

Timothy K. Liem, M.D.
Vascular Surgery Resident Physician, Department of Surgery, University of Missouri–Columbia, Columbia, Missouri

Donald Silver, M.D.
W. Alton Jones Distinguished Professor and Chairman, Department of Surgery, University of Missouri–Columbia, Columbia, Missouri

M ost physicians, especially cardiovascular surgeons, interventional radiologists, and cardiologists, use antithrombotic therapy or prophylaxis in their practice. Heparin and coumarin derivatives are the two anticoagulants most often prescribed. At times, patients requiring antithrombotic therapy may not be able to safely receive heparin or coumadin and the physician is required to use an alternative anticoagulant.

A variety of antithrombotic agents are currently available, awaiting approval by the Food and Drug Administration, undergoing clinical testing, or in development. These include low–molecular weight (LMW) heparins and heparinoids, direct thrombin inhibitors (hirudin, hirugen, hirulog, argatroban), defibrinogenating agents (ancrod, reptilase), and platelet function inhibitors (aspirin, ticlopidine, glycoprotein [GP] IIb/IIIa inhibitors).

This chapter will review the pharmacology, indications for use, and complications of the rapid-acting anticoagulants (e.g., heparin and heparin-related agents), sodium warfarin, and the platelet function inhibitors. Some of the newer thromboinhibitors (e.g., hirudin, hirugen, D-Phe-Pro-ArgCH$_2$Cl [PPACK], hirulog, argatroban) and defibrinogenating agents are briefly reviewed. Occasionally, physicians use fibrinolytic agents as anticoagulants. This occurs infrequently, and the fibrinolytic agents will not be reviewed in this chapter.

Advances in Vascular Surgery®, vol. 5
©1997, Mosby–Year Book, Inc.

201

HEPARIN AND HEPARIN-LIKE ANTICOAGULANTS

PHYSICAL PROPERTIES AND MECHANISMS OF ACTION

Unfractionated Heparin

Unfractionated heparins (UHs) with molecular weights ranging from 4,000 to 40,000 d, are glycosaminoglycans of varying length composed of repetitive disaccharide units (uronic acid and glucosamine). These disaccharide units have various carboxyl and sulfate substitutions that are responsible for the highly negative charge of heparin. Unfractionated heparins are derived primarily from bovine lung and porcine intestinal mucosa.

Low–Molecular Weight Heparins

Low-molecular weight heparins are derived from the enzymatic or alkaline degradation of UF benzyl esters purified from porcine intestinal mucosa. The average molecular weight of the various LMW heparin preparations ranges from 4,000 to 6,000 d.

Heparinoids

Danaparoid (Orgaran, Organon Inc., West Orange, NJ) is the most widely tested heparinoid. It is composed of heparan sulfate (83%), dermatan sulfate (12%), and chondroitin sulfate (5%). Like LMW heparin, danaparoid is derived from animal intestinal mucosa. It has a mean molecular weight of 6,000 d. Danaparoid is not yet approved for use in the United States. However, it may be obtained as a compassionate-use medication, usually in patients with heparin-induced thrombocytopenia (HIT).

Mechanisms of Action

Heparin binds to antithrombin III (AT III) in a 1:1 ratio via a specific pentasaccharide sequence that is present in only 30% of unfractionated and LMW heparin molecules. This causes a conformational change in AT III that exposes an active site for the neutralization of numerous activated plasma coagulation factors. Unfractionated and LMW heparins with the pentasaccharide sequence inactivate factor Xa via this mechanism. In contrast, thrombin inactivation requires the formation of a ternary complex in which thrombin and AT III bind simultaneously to heparin molecules with at least 18 to 20 saccharide units. Only 25% to 50% of the heparin molecules in the various LMW heparin preparations contain this critical length. Thus LMW heparins have reduced antithrombin activity while maintaining anti-Xa activity.

The heparan sulfate component of danaparoid also binds to AT III via the specific pentasaccharide sequence. The majority of its antithrombotic effect is through preferential inactivation of factor

Xa. The dermatan sulfate component of danaparoid also has slight anti-IXa activity, through a mechanism involving heparin co-factor II.

A recently discovered second mechanism of action for heparin has been elucidated. Tissue factor pathway inhibitor (TFPI) is a serine protease inhibitor produced by endothelial cells and hepatocytes. Although TFPI is present in minute amounts during baseline conditions, heparin causes a twofold to sixfold increase in TFPI via release from the endothelial surface. Unfractionated heparin may cause a greater degree of TFPI release than does LMW heparin. Tissue factor pathway inhibitor forms a complex with factor Xa, factor VIIa, and tissue factor and prevents the conversion of factor IX to IXa and factor X to Xa, thus preventing coagulation.

PHARMACOKINETICS
Unfractionated heparin binds to numerous plasma proteins, including platelet factor 4, vitronectin, fibronectin, and von Willebrand factor. It also binds to platelet GP Ib receptors and vascular endothelium. This may be responsible for the variable bioavailability and anticoagulant activity of UH. Heparin is cleared primarily via rapidly saturable binding to reticuloendothelial cells. If the plasma concentration exceeds this saturable limit, heparin is excreted slowly via the kidneys in a nonsaturable fashion. This results in a plasma half-life that is dose dependent and ranges from about 45 to 150 minutes for UH. The half-life of LMW heparin is approximately two to three times longer than that of UH. Renal failure and hepatic insufficiency have minimal effects on the clearance of heparin and LMW heparins. However, liver failure may affect the production of clotting factors and naturally occurring anticoagulant proteins (AT III, protein C, protein S).

Low–molecular weight heparins may have antithrombotic activity superior to that of UH. They also have greater bioavailability in plasma than UH does because of decreased binding to plasma proteins and vascular endothelium. As a result, weight-adjusted doses may be administered without therapeutic monitoring. Low–molecular weight heparins may be more effective antithrombotic agents because they also neutralize clot-bound factor Xa, unlike UH. The longer half-life of some LMW heparins allows once-daily administration. Low–molecular weight heparins and heparinoids are associated with a decreased risk of bleeding when compared with UH. This may be caused by a decrease in idiosyncratic platelet binding that occurs in as many as 30% of patients receiving UH.

ADMINISTRATION AND MONITORING

For rapid antithrombotic therapy, UH is administered intravenously in a loading dose of 100 units/kg and then at approximately 800 to 1,000 units/hr. We administer larger loading doses of 150 to 200 units/kg for patients with acute limb ischemia, iliofemoral venous thrombosis, and pulmonary embolism. We attempt to maintain the activated partial thromboplastin time (aPTT) at 1.6 to 2.0 times control. The aPTT is monitored every 6 hours for the first several days of therapy until the UH dosage and therapeutic response are stabilized.

Anticardiolipin antibodies, including lupus anticoagulants, prolong the phospholipid-dependent in vitro clotting tests, including the aPTT, prothrombin time (PT), dilute Russell's viper venom test, and kaolin clotting test. Antithrombotic therapy in patients with these antibodies may be regulated by measurement of heparin levels through protamine titration (therapeutic levels are greater than 0.2 unit/mL) or by using chromogenic anti–factor Xa assays (therapeutic levels are greater than 0.3 unit/mL).

Patients who undergo cardiopulmonary bypass require greater levels of UH anticoagulation (approximately 5 units/mL), a range where the aPTT is not reliable. In these circumstances, heparin therapy may be monitored by using the activated clotting time. Other alternatives to regulate heparin therapy include the whole blood clotting time (two to three times control), whole blood activated recalcification time (two to three times control), and calcium thrombin time (two to six times control).

We monitor the platelet count on a daily basis while the patient is receiving heparin therapy to allow early detection of HIT. If the platelet count decreases below 100,000/mL or decreases significantly (greater than 20%), we test for the presence of heparin-associated antibodies with platelet aggregation assays.

Patients with heterozygous AT III deficiency have approximately 50% to 60% of normal activity AT III. Antithrombin III–deficient patients with thrombotic episodes are treated with heparin. The occasional AT III–deficient patient who is particularly resistant to heparin therapy may require AT III concentrate. The dosage can be calculated by using the following formula:

$$\text{units required (IU)} = \frac{[\text{desired} - \text{baseline ATIII level}] \times \text{weight (kg)}}{1.4}$$

Antithrombin III concentrates may be used as an adjunct to heparin therapy in acute thrombotic events and as thrombotic prophylaxis for AT III–deficient patients in high-risk situations, e.g., parturition, surgery. The target range for the therapeutic administration of AT III concentrates is to obtain at least 80% of normal AT III activity.

Low–molecular weight heparin may be given as either a fixed dose or a weight-adjusted dose regimen. Low–molecular weight heparin antithrombotic prophylaxis or therapy does not routinely require laboratory monitoring. Danaparoid administered subcutaneously is readily absorbed and reaches peak anti-Xa activity within 4 to 5 hours. The dose and route of administration of danaparoid depend on the indications for use. As prophylaxis against thromboembolism, danaparoid is administered at 750 units twice daily subcutaneously. For rapid anticoagulation, it is administered as an IV bolus of 2,500 units with subsequent continuous infusion. The antithrombotic effect does not require routine monitoring.

THROMBOEMBOLISM PROPHYLAXIS

The risk of perioperative deep vein thrombosis (DVT) depends on the number of risk factors present. These include age greater than 40 years, obesity, malignancy, immobility, prior venous thromboembolism, varicose veins, low cardiac output, major trauma, and oral contraceptive use. The incidence of DVT ranges from 25% to 33% in patients undergoing general surgical procedures and 45% to 70% in patients having total hip replacement.[1] Thromboembolic complications are also more frequent in patients having other orthopedic procedures and in patients with multiple trauma.

Fixed low-dose UH prophylaxis (5,000 units SC every 8 or 12 hours) reduces the incidence of DVT in moderate and high-risk general surgery patients from approximately 25% to 8%.[2] The incidence of pulmonary embolism is reduced as well. However, fixed low-dose UH prophylaxis is not as effective in patients with hip fractures or in patients undergoing total hip or knee replacement. The efficacy of UH in some orthopedic patients may be improved by using an *adjusted* dose regimen that prolongs the aPTT 2 to 5 seconds above control. The aPTT is usually determined 2 to 6 hours after the first daily administration. Orthopedic and very high-risk general surgical patients are better served with other methods of thromboembolism prophylaxis such as oral warfarin, LMW heparin, adjusted-dose heparin, or combination prophylaxis (low-dose UH with intermittent pneumatic compression).

The duration of therapy should be tailored to the individual circumstance. Patients undergoing hip or knee replacements may be at increased risk of venous thromboembolism for greater than 3 to 5 weeks. Antithrombotic prophylaxis should be continued at least until the patient is fully ambulatory. Patients with spinal cord injuries and prolonged immobilization may require therapy for up to 3 months.

THERAPY FOR VENOUS THROMBOEMBOLISM

Intravenous heparin is effective initial therapy for patients with DVT. This has been verified in a recent randomized controlled trial comparing anticoagulation with heparin and acenocoumarol vs. acenocoumarol alone. Patients treated with heparin and the coumarin derivative had a significantly decreased incidence of proximal DVT extension and recurrent venous thromboembolism (20% vs. 6.7%).[3] We administer heparin as a bolus (100 to 200 units/kg intravenously) followed by a continuous IV infusion to obtain an aPTT between 1.6 and 2.0 times normal.

The optimal duration of heparin therapy has not been resolved. Treatment with 5 days of IV heparin has been demonstrated to be as effective as 10 days for the initial treatment of proximal vein thrombosis.[4] Both groups of patients were also treated with oral warfarin therapy for 12 weeks. We begin oral warfarin on the second day of IV heparin therapy. Heparin is continued until the PT has been in the desired range (International Normalization Ratio [INR] in the 2.0 to 3.0 range) for 2 consecutive days. This approach usually requires at least 5 days of heparin therapy.

Multicenter randomized controlled trials have evaluated outpatient LMW heparin as initial therapy for proximal vein thrombosis. In the largest of these studies, the incidence of recurrent thromboembolism in patients treated with conventional IV UH or SC LMW heparin was 6.7% and 5.3%, respectively.[5] The incidence of hemorrhagic complications was also comparable (1% and 2%). Based on the findings of this and similar studies, LMW heparin may become the preferred initial therapy for some patients with proximal vein thrombosis. Further investigation is warranted to identify which patients may be at increased risk for bleeding complications (e.g., ulcer diathesis, perioperative patients, liver failure, thrombocytopenia) and proximal extension of thromboembolism.

COMPLICATIONS

The most common nonhemorrhagic complication of UH therapy is HIT. Heparin-induced thrombocytopenia type I is caused by idiosyncratic, clinically insignificant platelet aggregation in the presence of heparin that is not immune mediated. Type II HIT is caused by IgG and IgM antibodies specific for heparin. Type II HIT occurs in approximately 3% to 5% of patients receiving UH therapy. Low–molecular weight heparin is associated with a decreased incidence of HIT when compared with UH.

The heparin-immunoglobulin complex causes platelet activation, the release reaction, and platelet aggregation. Antibodies can usually be detected by days 4 to 15 of heparin therapy and may persist for years. Type II HIT usually includes the triad of decreasing platelet count, resistance to anticoagulation with heparin, and new or progressive thromboembolic events while receiving heparin.

Heparin-induced thrombocytopenia antibodies may be detected with platelet aggregation or ^{14}C-serotonin release assays. The most sensitive and specific assay is the ^{14}C-serotonin release assay, but it is quite labor-intensive and requires several hours to perform. If proper platelet donors and heparin test concentrations are used, platelet aggregation assays have a comparable sensitivity (88%) and specificity (82% to 100%).

Management of type II HIT includes discontinuation of heparin therapy and use of alternative anticoagulants. Warfarin has been used with success but requires several days to achieve full anticoagulation. In the interim, LMW heparins or heparinoids may be

---

TABLE 1.

Cross-Reactivity of Heparin-Associated Antibodies With Low–Molecular Weight Heparins and Heparinoids

LMW heparin	
Mono-Embolex NM	60.8% (31/51)*
Dalteparin (Fragmin)	25.5% (13/51)*
Enoxaparin	34% (43/126)†
LMW heparinoid	
Danaparoid (Orgaran)	19.6% (10/51)*

*Data from Kikta MJ, Keller MP, Humphrey PW, et al: Can low molecular weight heparins and heparinoids be safely given to patients with heparin-induced thrombocytopenia syndrome? *Surgery* 114:705–710, 1993.
†Data from Slocum MM, Adams JG, Teel R, et al: The use of enoxaparin in patients with the heparin-induced thrombocytopenia syndrome. *J Vasc Surg* 23:839–843, 1996.

used if the heparin-associated antibody does not cross-react with these agents. The cross-reactivity rate with LMW heparin varies from 20% to 61%, depending on the commercial preparation.[6, 7] Table 1 presents a list of the cross-reactivity rates of some LMW heparin and heparinoid preparations.

Experience with the use of other alternative anticoagulants is limited in patients with HIT who require continued anticoagulation. Aspirin, dipyridamole, and dextran have provided minimal effectiveness as antithrombotic agents in patients with HIT. Other antithrombotic agents (e.g., hirudin, ancrod, argatroban) and potent platelet function inhibiting agents (GP IIb/IIIa inhibitors) are being evaluated in the management of patients with the HIT syndrome. We have found that HIT thromboses are relatively resistant to lysis with urokinase.

COUMARIN DERIVATIVES

VITAMIN K AND WARFARIN

Vitamin K is a coenzyme for the γ-carboxylation of glutamine (Glu) residues on coagulation factors II, VII, IX, and X and the natural anticoagulants protein C and protein S. The liver processes vitamin K according to the cycle shown in Figure 1. Vitamin K is first converted to its hydroquinone form (KH_2) via a reduced nicotinamide adenine dinucleotide phosphate–dependent reaction. During the conversion of Glu to γ-carboxyglutamate (Gla), vitamin KH_2 is oxidized into vitamin K epoxide. Continued γ-carboxylation of Glu requires that vitamin K be converted back to the KH_2 form via dithiol-dependent reactions. Each molecule of vitamin K is recycled several hundred (or even several thousand) times before it is degraded into inactive metabolites.[8]

Coumarin derivatives, including warfarin, block the conversion of vitamin K epoxide back to vitamin KH_2. This results in the production of vitamin K–dependent proteins that have a decreased number of Gla residues and decreased enzymatic activity. A decrease in the number of Gla residues from the usual 10 to 13 to 6 reduces coagulation factor biological activity by more than 95%.

An antithrombotic state depends on the natural degradation of functional coagulation factors present in the circulation and their replacement with the altered coagulation proteins. The half-lives of the vitamin K–dependent proteins are listed in Table 2. Factor VII and protein C have the shortest half-lives, approximately 6 hours, and factor II and factor X have longer half-lives of approximately 72 and 36 hours, respectively. Although warfarin may pro-

The Vitamin K Cycle

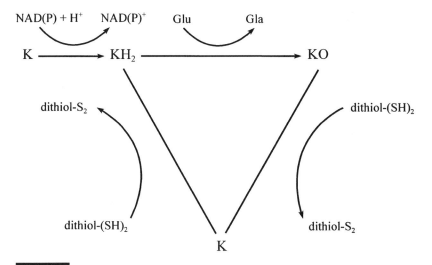

FIGURE 1.

The vitamin K cycle. Warfarin and other coumarin derivatives block the dithiol-dependent reactions decreasing the amount of the hydroquinone form of vitamin K *(KH₂)* available. *Abbreviations: K,* vitamin K; *NADP,* nicotinamide adenine dinucleotide phosphate; *KO,* vitamin K epoxide. (Courtesy of Liem T, Silver D: Coumadin: Principles of use. *Semin Vasc Surg,* 9:354–361, 1996.

long the PT within 24 hours of administration because of factor VII depletion, an antithrombotic state is not usually attained for 2 to 4 days.

Orally ingested warfarin is rapidly absorbed and reaches a maximum plasma concentration within 2 to 12 hours. Ninety-seven percent of warfarin circulates bound to albumin. The unbound portion is responsible for the anticoagulant effect. Warfarin has a half-life in the blood of approximately 36 to 42 hours. The amount of warfarin required to cause prolongation of the PT depends on the amount of dietary vitamin K, the age of the patient, and co-morbid conditions (liver failure, obstructive jaundice, starvation). Foods high in vitamin K derivatives (spinach, broccoli, cabbage, cow's milk, and yogurt) may make patients more resistant to the action of warfarin.

Numerous medications have also been found to potentiate or interfere with the activity of warfarin. Some of these are listed in

TABLE 2.
Plasma Half-Lives
of Vitamin
K–Dependent
Proteins

Factor II	72 hr
Factor VII	6 hr
Factor IX	24 hr
Factor X	36 hr
Protein C	6 hr
Protein S	72–96 hr

(Courtesy of Liem T, Silver D: Coumadin: Principles of use. *Semin Vasc Surg*, 9:354-361, 1996.)

Table 3. Patients receiving long-term oral anticoagulation who begin or stop taking a medication that may interfere with or potentiate warfarin activity should be monitored with more frequent PT measurements.

INITIATING WARFARIN THERAPY

Warfarin therapy is initiated by the oral intake of 5 to 10 mg/day. Reduced dosages should be given to elderly patients, patients with liver disease, and those with vitamin K deficiency (malnutrition, long-term parenteral nutrition). Because factor II and factor X depletion may take 2 to 4 days, heparin should be administered during the first few days of warfarin therapy for patients in whom immediate anticoagulation is necessary. Warfarin may cause a transient thrombophilic state because of depletion of protein C before depletion of factors II, IX, and X.[8] This is particularly true for patients with protein C deficiency, in whom there is a significant risk of warfarin-induced skin necrosis. Concomitant heparin administration (5,000 units subcutaneously every 8 hours for 3 to 4 days) decreases the risk of this complication.

Patients beginning warfarin therapy as an outpatient for indications such as atrial fibrillation and perioperative DVT prophylaxis may usually receive lower doses of warfarin safely without concomitant heparin administration.

TABLE 3.

Drug Interactions With Oral Anticoagulants

Potentiate	Antagonize
Allopurinol	Antihistamines
Aminoglycosides	Carbamazepine
Anabolic steroids	Cholestyramine
Chloramphenicol	Glutethimide
Chlorpromazine	Griseofulvin
Cimetidine	Haloperidol
Clofibrate	Oral contraceptives
Cotrimoxazole	Phenobarbital
Dipyridamole	Phenytoin
Disulfiram	Spironolactone
Metronidazole	Vitamin K
Phenylbutazone	
Quinidine	
Oral hypoglycemic drugs	
Salicylates	
Tricyclic antidepressants	

(Courtesy of Humphrey PR, Hoch JR, Silver D: hemostasis and thrombosis, in Moore WS (ed): *Vascular Surgery: A Comprehensive Review,* ed 4. Philadelphia, WB Saunders, 1993.)

MONITORING WARFARIN THERAPY

The PT is most commonly used to monitor warfarin therapy. This test is sensitive to changes in activity of factors II, VII, IX, and X. The PT is performed by adding thromboplastin (tissue factor and phospholipid derived from lung, heart, or brain tissue) and calcium to citrated plasma. Thromboplastins vary according to their ability to activate the external coagulation cascade and are graded by the International Sensitivity Index (ISI). The INR attempts to standardize PT assays that use different thromboplastins according to the following equation:

$$INR = [\text{Patient prothrombin time (sec)/Population prothrombin time (sec)}]^{ISI}$$

The PT should be monitored on a daily basis for the first 4 to 5 days of warfarin therapy. The INR usually achieves the desired range during this period. A longer period of daily monitoring will be required in patients resistant to warfarin. Once the therapeutic range is attained, the PT can be monitored two to three times per week and, when stable, every 4 to 6 weeks.

Many patients are receiving heparin when warfarin therapy is initiated. Concomitant administration of heparin prolongs the PT because of the inactivation of factors IIa, IXa, and Xa by AT III. It should be expected that the PT will decrease when heparin treatment is discontinued. The effect of heparin on the PT can be reduced by removing the heparin from the test plasma or by stopping the heparin infusion 4 to 6 hours before obtaining blood for the PT.

Other methods have been proposed in attempts to improve monitoring of the external coagulation cascade in patients receiving warfarin. These include radioimmunoassays for Gla-containing factor II and assays for the individual vitamin K–dependent factors. An enzyme-linked coagulation assay detects inactivation of the extrinsic pathway via a method that is not affected by concurrent heparin administration. These tests have not gained wide acceptance.

THROMBOEMBOLISM PROPHYLAXIS

Warfarin effectively prevents venous thromboembolism. The incidence of clinical venous thrombosis in patients with hip fractures was decreased from 28.7% in the control group to 2.7% in the group receiving oral anticoagulants.[9] Other studies confirm the benefit of warfarin prophylaxis in orthopedic and gynecologic surgical patients. Warfarin should be initiated the evening before surgery or as early as possible postoperatively. The INR should be in the 2.0 to 3.0 range. The optimal duration of warfarin therapy has not been established, but it is usually continued until the patient has resumed usual activities. The increased risk of venous thromboembolism may persist as long as 3 to 5 weeks postoperatively.

Low-dose warfarin (1 mg/day) decreases thrombosis in cancer patients with long-term venous access catheters,[10] but it is ineffective as prophylaxis in orthopedic patients. Because of the potential for hemorrhage, warfarin use should be limited to surgical patients at high risk for thrombotic complications (e.g., recent femur or hip fractures, hip surgery, prior venous thromboembolism, certain malignancies that induce a prothrombotic state).

MANAGEMENT OF VENOUS THROMBOLISM

Standard treatment for venous thrombosis and pulmonary embolism includes long-term warfarin therapy. An INR of 2.0 to 3.0 is as effective as more intensive therapy (INR of 3.0 to 4.5) in reducing the risk of recurrent thromboembolism, and it is also associated with a decreased risk of hemorrhagic complications.

The duration of therapy should be tailored to the circumstances surrounding the venous thromboembolism. Patients with irreversible risk factors (malignancy, prior venous thrombosis, congenital hypercoagulable states) or those with idiopathic venous thromboembolism have higher risks of recurrence than do patients with reversible risk factors (postoperative patients). Four weeks of warfarin may be adequate in patients with transient risk factors, whereas 3 or more months is necessary in patients with permanent risk factors. We treat patients with venous thromboembolism for a minimum of 3 months, usually 6 months. Patients with recurrent venous thromboembolism are treated for 6 to 12 months. Patients with congenital hypercoagulable states and thromboembolism are treated for life.

PERIPHERAL VASCULAR DISEASE

The role of warfarin in patients with atherosclerotic peripheral vascular disease is not as clear. Warfarin has been used in patients with arterial thromboembolic events to decrease the risk of recurrence. It has also been used to decrease the incidence of graft failure in patients with infrainguinal arterial reconstructions. Two randomized trials found that warfarin significantly decreased the incidence of graft failure in patients with infrainguinal arterial reconstructions,[11, 12] whereas other studies found no decrease in graft thrombosis with warfarin.[13] Our practice is to offer warfarin (INR of 2.0 to 3.0) in combination with aspirin to patients with synthetic infrainguinal bypass grafts. Warfarin may also have a role in some patients with prior graft failure in whom secondary graft patency has been restored. Warfarin has an important role in patients with some hypercoagulable states and grafts.

COMPLICATIONS

The major complication of warfarin therapy is hemorrhage. The true incidence of bleeding is probably more accurately reflected in observational and population-based studies (3% to 12% per year) than in well-monitored clinical trials. The usual sites of major hemorrhage include the gastrointestinal tract, retroperitoneum, extremities, pelvic organs, and CNS.

The risk factors for bleeding complications associated with oral anticoagulation include the intensity of warfarin therapy, the age of the patient, and the type of coumarin derivative used. More intense anticoagulation (INR of 3.0 to 4.5) is associated with a greater incidence of bleeding (22% vs. 4%) than less intense warfarin therapy (INR of 2.0).[14] Minor hemorrhagic events are not reliable indicators that major bleeding is likely to occur.

Patient characteristics that are also associated with an increased risk of hemorrhage include increasing age, a history of gastrointestinal bleeding, hypertension, cerebrovascular disease, heart disease, renal failure, and the presence of malignancy. The greatest likelihood of bleeding occurs during the first months of therapy. Increased bleeding events may occur when warfarin dosages are adjusted (e.g., in the perioperative period) or when vitamin K intake changes significantly (dietary modifications, critical illness). Bleeding, which occurs in the presence of an INR of 5.0 or less, may have other associated causes (e.g., peptic ulcer disease, malignancy).

Other less common complications include alopecia, urticaria, dermatitis, fever, nausea, diarrhea, abdominal cramping, and hypersensitivity reactions. Warfarin-induced skin necrosis is a rare complication that occurs in 0.01% to 0.1% of patients receiving warfarin. The incidence increases to approximately 3% in protein C–deficient patients initiating warfarin therapy. Necrosis may even occur in patients who had previously tolerated oral anticoagulation.

The mechanism of warfarin-induced skin necrosis may involve the depletion of protein C before reductions in the other vitamin K–dependent proteins. This causes a temporary thrombophilic state, which may lead to dermal venous thrombosis. The most likely sites of dermal venous thrombosis are the breast, thigh, or buttocks, although other areas with increased subcutaneous fat may also be involved. Dermal venous thrombosis occurs more often with larger loading doses of warfarin, although this is not clearly established. We recommend that heparin be administered concurrent with the first 3 to 5 days of warfarin to decrease the likelihood of skin necrosis.

Warfarin should be avoided during pregnancy because of possible teratogenic effects on the fetus. Craniofacial and bony anomalies may occur with warfarin exposure in the first trimester; CNS anomalies may occur in the third trimester. If thrombosis prophylaxis or therapy is required during pregnancy, we prefer unfractionated or LMW heparin. Neither of these medications cross the placenta.

REVERSAL OF WARFARIN ANTICOAGULATION
The optimal methods by which warfarin anticoagulation is reversed depend on the amount of INR prolongation and whether the patient is bleeding. Hirsh and colleagues have formulated recom-

mendations as follows[15]: if the INR is less than 6.0 and the patient is not bleeding, the next few doses should be omitted and warfarin restarted at a lower dose. If the INR is between 6.0 and 10.0 and the patient is not bleeding, vitamin K (1 to 2 mg subcutaneously) can be administered. If the INR is greater than 10.0 and the patient is not bleeding, higher doses of vitamin K (3 to 10 mg subcutaneously) can be given. Additional doses of vitamin K are indicated if the INR is still significantly prolonged in 6 to 12 hours. If the INR is greater than 20.0 or the patient has significant bleeding, vitamin K (10 mg subcutaneously or intravenously) should be administered in combination with fresh frozen plasma or prothrombin complex concentrate.[15]

Elective surgery and invasive diagnostic procedures in patients receiving warfarin should be delayed if possible until the oral anticoagulation can be discontinued safely. If the patient requires continued anticoagulation or the surgical/diagnostic procedure cannot be delayed, there are options regarding the management of these patients. Our first choice is to discontinue warfarin therapy 4 to 5 days before surgery. Heparin is administered at a therapeutic level during this time, discontinued 3 to 6 hours before surgery, and reinstituted after surgery. Alternatively, the warfarin dosage is reduced to allow the INR to reach low therapeutic or subtherapeutic levels. The choice depends on the original indication for anticoagulation and the type of surgical procedure being performed. Patients receiving warfarin who require emergent surgery can have the anticoagulation reversed with vitamin K (10 mg IV) and/or fresh frozen plasma if fluid volume is not a problem. It is easier to "reanticoagulate" the patient if fresh frozen plasma has been used.

Patients with mitral or combined mechanical valve replacements have a significant incidence of thromboembolic complications when warfarin therapy is discontinued in the perioperative period. A protocol that replaces warfarin with heparin may be beneficial in reducing these complications. Discontinuation of warfarin treatment 3 to 5 days before noncardiac surgery (without heparin replacement) in patients with aortic valve prostheses appears to be associated with a low incidence of thromboembolism.

Patients who are to undergo relatively minor procedures in which mechanical hemostasis can be achieved without difficulty do not need full reversal of warfarin anticoagulation. Although the incidence of bleeding after dental procedures is greater when warfarin therapy is not discontinued, local measures to obtain hemostasis are usually successful. Tranexamic acid mouthwash, an antifibrinolytic agent, has been used to reduce bleeding after oral surgery in patients receiving warfarin.

PLATELET FUNCTION INHIBITORS
ASPIRIN

Aspirin irreversibly acetylates cyclooxygenase (prostaglandin H synthase) and inhibits the conversion of platelet and endothelial arachidonic acid to thromboxane A_2 and prostacyclin, respectively. This effect lasts for the life span of the platelet, whereas the endothelium may generate new cyclooxygenase. Low doses of aspirin (80 mg/day) are as effective as larger doses of aspirin in inhibiting thromboxane A_2 generation. Daily antiplatelet therapy is required to maintain this benefit because there is a daily turnover of approximately 10% of the circulating platelets.

The Antiplatelet Trialists' Collaboration reviewed the efficacy of aspirin in the prevention of thrombotic complications in more than 100,000 patients. In high-risk patients, aspirin reduced the incidence of nonfatal myocardial infarction by 30%, nonfatal stroke by 30%, and vascular death by 17%.[16] This risk reduction may not apply to patients at low risk for cardiovascular complications. In addition, the benefits of aspirin must be weighed against a possible increased risk of hemorrhagic stroke.

Peripheral vascular disease is a good indicator of atherosclerotic disease elsewhere and places the patient at increased risk for myocardial infarction and ischemic stroke. We recommend lifelong aspirin (80 to 325 mg/day) to all patients with atherosclerotic peripheral vascular disease unless there is a contraindication. They are advised to take the aspirin with meals to reduce the incidence of gastric irritation and ulceration. There may be some benefit in the prevention of peripheral arterial thromboembolism. We offer aspirin and low-intensity warfarin (INR of 2.0 to 3.0) to patients with synthetic infrainguinal grafts. The incidence of bleeding complications may increase slightly depending on the intensity of aspirin and warfarin therapy.

TICLOPIDINE

Ticlopidine inhibits the binding of fibrinogen to the platelet GP IIb/IIIa receptor, the primary receptor involved in platelet aggregation. It reduces the incidence of stroke, myocardial infarction, and vascular death by as much as 23% in various patients with atherosclerosis.[17] Ticlopidine is administered orally in a dose of 250 mg twice per day. Side effects of ticlopidine include a 2% incidence of reversible agranulocytosis, neutropenia, and pancytopenia. Ticlopidine may be used as an alternative in patients who are unable to tolerate or have contraindications to aspirin.

GLYCOPROTEIN IIB/IIIA INHIBITORS

Fibrinogen, fibrin, von Willebrand factor, and fibronectin have recognition specificity for the platelet GP IIb/IIIa receptor through the amino acid sequence Arg-Gly-Asp (RGD). The first GP IIb/IIIa inhibitor to be made commercially available was c7E3 (abciximab, Eli Lilly and Company), the Fab fragment of a murine monoclonal antibody directed against the GP IIb/IIIa receptor. Subsequently, naturally occurring proteins (trigramin) containing the RGD sequence have been isolated from the venom of several species of vipers. Most recently, synthetic RGD and KGD (Lys-Gly-Asp) analogues (MK-852, Merck; G4120, Genentech; Integrelin, COR Therapeutics) have been manufactured and have undergone clinical trials.

Abciximab, Integrelin, and several other GP IIb/IIIa inhibitors were found to decrease ischemic complications in patients undergoing coronary angioplasty, patients with unstable angina, and patients with acute myocardial infarctions.[18] An orally absorbable formulation is under development for long-term platelet function inhibition. Future indications for GP IIb/IIIa inhibitors may include cerebrovascular, aortoiliac, and infrainguinal disease. The administration of GP IIb/IIIa inhibitors may also allow patients in whom heparin-associated antibodies develop to continue to receive heparin.[19]

DIRECT THROMBIN INHIBITORS

HIRUDIN

Hirudin is a 65–amino acid polypeptide derived from the salivary gland of the medicinal leech *(Hirudo medicinalis).* Hirudin and the more widely available recombinant hirudin have similar pharmacologic properties. They form a stoichiometric complex, with thrombin blocking the catalytic site, substrate groove, and anion binding site.[20] This prevents thrombin from catalyzing the formation of fibrin and factors Va, VIIIa, and XIIIa. Hirudin also inhibits thrombin-induced platelet activation and aggregation.

Hirudin may be administered via an IV or subcutaneous route. After an initial distribution phase, hirudin follows first-order elimination kinetics. It is excreted via glomerular filtration in its active form and has a half-life ranging from 1 to 2 hours. The aPTT, PT, and thrombin time (TT) are prolonged by the administration of hirudin. The dose-response curve obtained with the PT is not sensitive enough for clinical use, so the TT and aPTT are more commonly used to monitor hirudin therapy.

Numerous clinical trials have compared hirudin with heparin in the treatment of patients undergoing coronary angioplasty[21] and coronary thrombolysis[22] and in patients with unstable angina.[23] Hirudin was associated with a decreased risk of ischemic events when compared with heparin therapy.[21–23] Some trials also demonstrated an increased incidence of major hemorrhage, although this complication usually occurred when hirudin was given in conjunction with thrombolytic agents.[24] Hirudin has been used successfully as an alternative anticoagulant in patients with HIT.[25] As with heparin, hirudin has the potential to cause an immunologic reaction. Unlike heparin, however, no significant interactions have been found between hirudin and other blood proteins.[20] Hirudin is also characterized as a weak immunogen in animal and human studies. Future indications for hirudin may include venous thromboembolism prophylaxis and therapy, treatment for disseminated intravascular coagulation, and anticoagulation for cardiopulmonary bypass and hemodialysis.

HIRUGEN, ARGATROBAN, HIRULOG

Hirugen is a synthetic peptide fragment of hirudin specific for the anion binding exosite. It prevents the binding of thrombin to fibrinogen and platelet receptors. Because the active site of thrombin is not blocked, continued activity against smaller thrombin substrates may be present. D-Phe-Pro-ArgCH$_2$Cl and argatroban are synthetic inhibitors that bind to the active site of thrombin. The inhibitor PPACK binds irreversibly whereas argatroban is only a competitive inhibitor.

Hirulogs are a group of synthetic proteins derived from the combination of hirugen and PPACK-like substances. They are potent inhibitors of thrombin because they bind both the catalytic site and the anion binding exosite. Hirulogs have been compared with heparin in clinical trials of patients undergoing coronary thrombolysis.[26] They are at least as effective as heparin and are associated with a comparable hemorrhagic complication rate.

ANCROD

Ancrod is a 234–amino acid serine protease derived from the venom of the Malayan pit viper *(Calloselasma rhodostoma).* Ancrod cleaves fibrinopeptides A, AY, and AP from circulating fibrinogen. This results in a fibrin molecule that cannot undergo cross-linking and is susceptible to fibrinolysis by plasmin and phagocytosis by the reticuloendothelial system (RES). The reduced plasma concentration of fibrinogen also improves rheology by decreasing the viscosity of blood significantly. The circulating half-life of ancrod is 3 to 5 hours initially, followed by a longer elimination half-life of 9 to 12 hours when less than 10% of the initial dose remains. Ancrod is cleared by the RES; it is also excreted via the kidneys in its active form.

Ancrod may be administered via slow IV infusion or via SC injection. Fibrinogen levels in the range of 40 to 60 mg/dL are adequate for hemostasis and are effective in the prevention of spontaneous thromboses. Full antithrombotic therapy may be achieved by the administration of 70 to 100 units intravenously (1 to 2 units/kg) over a period of 12 to 36 hours. After the initial dose, ancrod, 1 to 2 units/kg/24 hr, is given intravenously or subcutaneously to maintain the fibrinogen level at 40 to 60 mg/dL. Plasma fibrinogen should be measured every 12 hours for the initial 48 hours and then daily. Ancrod may be used as prophylaxis against perioperative venous thromboembolism. The plasma fibrinogen concentration should be in the range of 40 to 60 mg/dL at the time of surgery. This requires administration the day before surgery because more than 12 hours may be required to attain an antithrombotic state.

Some patients with HIT who require continued anticoagulation have been treated successfully with ancrod. It also may be useful in patients with AT III deficiency and thromboembolic events who are resistant to heparin therapy. Other potential indications for ancrod include acute stroke, venous thromboembolism, anticoagulation for hemodialysis, cardiopulmonary bypass, and peripheral vascular surgery.

Ancrod therapy is associated with fever, allergic reactions, and the development of resistance. The latter complication occurs with the continued administration of ancrod for several weeks. Ancrod is contraindicated during pregnancy because of the potential for teratogenesis. Hemorrhagic complications are more likely to occur with decreasing plasma fibrinogen concentrations, especially when levels decrease to less than 20 mg/dL. Cessation of ancrod therapy will allow a return of the fibrinogen to normal within days. If uncontrollable bleeding is present, fibrinogen should be repleted with an infusion of cryoprecipitate.

Other natural anticoagulants and fibrinolytic agents derived from sources such as the hookworm, vampire bat saliva, sandfly, and *Ornithodoros* tick are under study. These nontraditional sources may contribute to our ability to successfully treat patients with antithrombotic therapy.

CONCLUSION

Unfractionated heparin and warfarin remain "standard therapy" for many patients with arterial and venous thromboembolic events. Alternative antithrombotic agents are available for the minority of patients in whom these agents are contraindicated. In addition, randomized clinical trials have demonstrated that these agents (e.g., LMW heparins, GP IIb/IIIa inhibitors, hirudin derivatives) may be effective and safe in selected patients.

REFERENCES

1. Silver D: An overview of venous thromboembolism prophylaxis. *Am J Surg* 161:537–540, 1991.
2. Clagett GP, Anderson FA Jr, Heit J, et al: Prevention of venous thromboembolism. *Chest* 108:312S–334S, 1995.
3. Brandjes DP, Heijboer H, Buller HR, et al: Acenocoumarol and heparin compared with acenocoumarol alone in the initial treatment of proximal vein thrombosis. *N Engl J Med* 327:1485–1489, 1992.
4. Hull RD, Raskob GE, Rosenbloom D, et al: Heparin for 5 days as compared with 10 days in the initial treatment of proximal venous thrombosis. *N Engl J Med* 322:1260–1264, 1990.
5. Levine M, Gent M, Hirsh J, et al: A comparison of low-molecular-weight heparin administered primarily at home with unfractionated heparin administered in the hospital for proximal deep-vein thrombosis. *N Engl J Med* 334:677–681, 1996.
6. Kikta MJ, Keller MP, Humphrey PW, et al: Can low molecular weight heparins and heparinoids be safely given to patients with heparin-induced thrombocytopenia syndrome? *Surgery* 114:705–710, 1993.
7. Slocum MM, Adams JG, Teel R, et al: Use of enoxaparin in patients with the heparin-induced thrombocytopenia syndrome. *J Vasc Surg* 23:839–843, 1996.
8. Vermeer C, Hamulyak K: Pathophysiology of vitamin K–deficiency and oral anticoagulants. *Thromb Haemost* 66:153–159, 1991.
9. Sevitt S, Gallagher NG: Prevention of venous thrombosis and pulmonary embolism in injured patients. *Lancet* 2:981–989, 1959.
10. Bern MM, Lokich JJ, Wallach SR, et al: Very low doses of warfarin can prevent thrombosis in central venous catheters. *Ann Intern Med* 112:423–428, 1990.
11. Kretschmer G, Wenzl E, Piza E, et al: The influence of anticoagulant treatment on the probability of function in femoropopliteal vein bypass surgery: Analysis of a clinical series (1970 to 1985) and interim evaluation of a controlled clinical trial. *Surgery* 102:453–459, 1987.
12. Kretschmer GJ, Holzenbein T: The role of anticoagulation in infrainguinal bypass surgery, in Yao JST, Pearce WH (eds): *The Ischemic Extremity: Advances in Treatment.* E Norwalk, Conn, Appleton & Lange, 1995, pp 447–454.

13. Arfidsson B, Lundgren F, Drott C, et al: Influence of coumarin treatment on patency and limb salvage after peripheral arterial reconstructive surgery. *Am J Surg* 159:556–560, 1990.

14. Hull R, Hirsh J, Jay R, et al: Different intensities of oral anticoagulant therapy in the treatment of proximal-vein thrombosis. *N Engl J Med* 307:1676–1681, 1982.

15. Hirsh J, Dalen JE, Deykin D, et al: Oral anticoagulants, mechanism of action, clinical effectiveness, and optimal therapeutic range. *Chest* 108:231S–246S, 1995.

16. Antiplatelet Trialists' Collaboration: Collaborative overview of randomized trials of antiplatelet therapy: I. Prevention of death, myocardial infarction, and stroke by prolonged antiplatelet therapy in various categories of patients. *BMJ* 308:81–106, 1994.

17. Gent M, Blakely JA, Easton JD, et al: The Canadian American Ticlopidine Study (CATS) in thromboembolic stroke. *Lancet* 2:1215–1220, 1989.

18. Lefkovits J, Plow EF, Topol EJ: Platelet glycoprotein IIb/IIIa receptors in cardiovascular medicine. *N Engl J Med* 332:1553–1559, 1995.

19. Liem TK, Teel R, Shukla S, et al: The glycoprotein IIb/IIIa antagonist c7E3 inhibits platelet aggregation in the presence of heparin associated antibodies. *J Vasc Surg* 25:124–130, 1997.

20. Markwardt F: Hirudin and derivatives as anticoagulant agents. *Thromb Haemost* 66:141–152, 1991.

21. Van den Bos AA, Deckers JW, Heyndrickx GR, et al: Safety and efficacy of recombinant hirudin (CGP 39 393) versus heparin in patients with stable angina undergoing coronary angioplasty. *Circulation* 88:2058–2066, 1993.

22. Cannon CP, McCabe CH, Henry TD, et al: A pilot trial of recombinant desulfatohirudin compared with heparin in conjunction with tissue-type plasminogen activator and aspirin for acute myocardial infarction: Results of the Thrombolysis in Myocardial Infarction (TIMI) 5 trial. *Am J Coll Cardiol* 23:993–1003, 1994.

23. Topol EJ, Fuster V, Harrington RA, et al: Recombinant hirudin for unstable angina pectoris: A multicenter, randomized angiographic trial. *Circulation* 89:1557–1566, 1994.

24. Global Use of Strategies to Open Coronary Arteries (GUSTO) IIa Investigators: Randomized trial of intravenous heparin versus recombinant hirudin for acute coronary syndromes. *Circulation* 90:1624–1630, 1994.

25. Nand S: Hirudin therapy for heparin-associated thrombocytopenia and deep venous thrombosis. *Am J Hematol* 43:310–311, 1993.

26. Lidon RM, Theroux P, Bonan R, et al: A pilot early angiographic patency study using a direct thrombin inhibitor as adjunctive therapy to streptokinase in acute myocardial infarction. *Circulation* 89:1567–1572, 1994.

CHAPTER 14

The Role of Growth Factors in Lower Extremity Ischemia and Nonhealing Wounds

Robert Y. Rhee, M.D.
Assistant Professor of Surgery, Section of Vascular Surgery, Department of Surgery, University of Pittsburgh School of Medicine, Pittsburgh, Pennsylvania

Marshall W. Webster, M.D.
Professor of Surgery and Chief, Section of Vascular Surgery, Department of Surgery, University of Pittsburgh School of Medicine, Pittsburgh, Pennsylvania

David L. Steed, M.D.
Professor of Surgery and Director, Wound Healing Clinic, Section of Vascular Surgery, Department of Surgery, University of Pittsburgh School of Medicine, Pittsburgh, Pennsylvania

W ound healing is the tissue response to injury and the subsequent reparative process. Despite significant advances in elucidation of the cellular and molecular biology of wound healing, a clear understanding of the critical and often multifactorial regulatory phenomena in wound healing is lacking. To simplify this continuous and complex process, the wound healing response can be divided into three distinct phases: *inflammation, fibroplasia, and maturation.*

Growth factors are polypeptides that control the growth, differentiation, and metabolism of tissue and bloodborne cells during each of the three phases of wound healing.[1] They are present throughout the body in only minute concentrations yet exert a powerful local influence on wound repair. Although the exact role of individual growth factors in normal wound healing is still not certain, in vitro growth factor activities have been well documented.

Growth factors are named for their tissue of origin (platelet-derived growth factor, [PDGF]), their biological action (transforming growth factor [TGF]), or the cell on which they act (epidermal growth factor [EGF])[2, 3] (Table 1). They have both paracrine (affecting adjacent cells) and autocrine (self-regulating) functions. Some growth factors are transported plasma bound to large carrier proteins and are thus delivered as endocrine factors. Generally, growth factors act by binding to cell surface receptors to stimulate cell growth.[3]

The platelet, which is critical to the initiation of wound healing, is a rich source of growth factors, including PDGF, TGF, and EGF.[4] Growth factors are chemoattractants for neutrophils, monocytes (macrophages), fibroblasts, and endothelial cells.[5] Although growth factors are initially released into the wound by the platelet, other cells begin growth factor production shortly after the initial wound healing process. Specifically, macrophages release po-

TABLE 1.

Summary of Growth Factors Involved in Wound Healing

Growth Factor	Source	Action
TGF-α	Platelets, macrophages, keratinocytes	Activates neutrophils; fibroblast mitogen; stimulates angiogenesis
TGF-β	Platelets, macrophages, lymphocytes	Stimulates fibroplasia, angiogenesis; induces proliferation of many different cells
PDGF	Platelets, macrophages, endothelial cells	Chemoattractant for neutrophils, fibroblasts; mitogen for smooth muscle cells and fibroblasts
FGF	Neutral tissue, nearly ubiquitous	Stimulates endothelial cell growth; mitogen for mesodermal and neuroectodermal-derived cells
EGF	Salivary gland	Mitogen for keratinocytes, endothelial cells, and fibroblasts
IGF	Liver	Mitogen for fibroblasts; stimulates smooth muscle cells, lymphocytes, chondrocytes

Abbreviations: TGF, transforming growth factor; *PDGF,* platelet-derived growth factor; *FGF,* fibroblast growth factor; *EGF,* epidermal growth factor; *IGF,* insulin-like growth factor.

tent growth factors such as tumor necrosis factor (TNF). Keratino-cyte proliferation can be stimulated by EGF, insulin-like growth factor type 1 (IGF-1), TGF, and interleukin-1 (IL-1). Wound remodeling may be controlled by collagenase production stimulated by EGF, TNF, IL-1, and PDGF.[4–6] Thus, it appears that all phases of wound healing are either directly or indirectly controlled by growth factors. It is with this premise that clinical trials involving the use of various growth factors in wound healing are born.

WOUND HEALING

When injury occurs to tissues, subendothelial parenchyma come into contact with blood components and initiate a hemostatic response.[4] The hemostatic response includes vasoconstriction, platelet activation, and coagulation.[5] When platelets are activated, they aggregate and initiate the clotting cascade, including both the intrinsic and extrinsic systems. The fibrinolytic system is also activated to prevent coagulation from extending beyond the margins of the wound.[5, 6] The kininogen and complement cascades are initiated as well. These cascades produce local vasoactive responses and alter capillary permeability.[6]

Simultaneously, via the same mediators, inflammation begins, along with an orderly migration of cells into the wound. Cells become activated and release cytokines that act as mitogens and chemoattractants. White blood cells enter the wound to phagocytize bacteria within the wound. Circulating monocytes enter the wound area to become tissue macrophages. These macrophages are important as phagocytes but also regulate cellular activities during the subsequent stages of wound healing. Fibroblasts enter the wound and rapidly proliferate to produce interstitial matrix proteins and collagen. Endothelial cells bud as the process of angiogenesis begins. After adequate granulation formation and epithelialization from wound edges, the final stage of wound healing occurs with contracture and remodeling.

INFLAMMATION

The inflammatory response is stimulated after injury. The goal of immediate vasoconstriction is to control local hemorrhage within the wound space.[5] Platelets are exposed to collagen within the vessel wall beneath the endothelium and aggregate to initiate coagulation. Serotonin and thromboxane are released to promote local vasoconstriction, which keeps locally acting growth factors within the wound space. However, vasodilation occurs shortly thereafter to allow healing factors to be brought into the wound. The vasodilatation is mediated by histamine, which is found in platelets, as well as mast cells and basophils. At the same time there is a local increase in vascular permeability that allows bloodborne factors to enter the wound.

Activation of the coagulation system amplifies the inflammatory response triggered by platelets. The intrinsic response of the coagulation cascade is activated by Hageman factor (factor XII) when it comes into contact with collagen. In the presence of high–molecular weight kininogen, a precursor of bradykinin and pre-kallikrein, factor XII activates factor XI, then factor IX and subsequently factor VIII. The extrinsic-system portion of the coagulation cascade is initiated by thromboplastin, which is formed from phospholipids and glycoproteins released when blood comes into contact with injured tissue. In the presence of calcium, factor VII is activated. Both the intrinsic and extrinsic systems can then activate the final common pathway leading to the formation of fibrin and fibrin polymerization.

Arachidonic acid is produced and serves as an intermediate for the production of prostaglandins, thromboxane, or leukotrienes. Prostaglandins are intense vasodilators that act in conjunction with histamine, bradykinin, and components of the complement system to increase vascular permeability. Thromboxane causes platelet aggregation and vasoconstriction.[5]

The complement cascade is also activated by platelets. In addition, neutral proteases activate portions of the complement systems. The final common pathway of complement cascade activity leads to the formation of C5a and C3a. These powerful anaphylotoxins cause degranulation of mast cells and histamine release, as well as being potent vasodilators. They lead to the margination and intravascular aggregation of white blood cells and cause adherence to vascular endothelium and entry into the wound. C5a is significantly more potent than C3a, but C3a is present in much higher concentrations.

The neutrophil enters the wound to phagocytize bacteria. Neutrophils are not necessary for wound healing in that wounds can heal in animals when neutrophils are depleted. However, without white blood cells, the probability of infection is increased. Factors released by the inflammatory process act as chemoattractants for neutrophils. Activated neutrophils release free oxygen radicals and lysosomal enzymes, including neutral proteases, elastase, and collagenase, which aid in host defense. The neutrophils themselves are removed by tissue macrophages.

The tissue macrophage has migrated into the wound by the third day and serves as the principal cell regulating wound healing. This cell is essential to wound healing and wounds cannot heal without it. The macrophage differentiates into either an inflammatory macrophage or a responsive macrophage. The macrophage regulates degradation of extracellular connective tissue by enzyme secretion and phagocytosis. It also regulates matrix remodeling. Growth factors such as PDGF and TGF, as well as interleukins and TNF, are subsequently produced by macrophages.

Extracellular matrix is composed of proteins embedded in a polysaccharide gel secreted by fibroblasts. Some of these proteins, such as collagen or elastin, are important for wound structure, and others, such as fibronectin or laminin, promote cell adhesion. The polysaccharide gel is composed of glycosaminoglycans coupled with proteoglycans. They allow nutrients to diffuse into cells and hold the cellular structure together. Adhesion proteins keep the cells adhering to the matrix. Fibronectin is an adhesion molecule that encourages cell surface adhesion, as do thrombospondin, von Willebrand factor, and laminin. Fibronectin is a strong opsonin and a chemoattractant for circulating monocytes and acts to stimulate differentiation of monocytes to active tissue macrophages.

FIBROPLASIA

Fibroplasia begins as macrophages and then fibroblasts proliferate in the wound while the number of neutrophils decreases. This begins the process of matrix formation, including collagen synthesis. At the same time, angiogenesis begins, followed by wound contracture and epithelialization. At this stage the inflammatory response is halted because inflammatory mediators are no longer produced and the mediators already present are inactivated. Mediators can also be removed from the wound by diffusion or by wound macrophages. Neutrophils are reduced by lessening the number entering into the wound. Fibroplasia begins about 5 days after injury and may continue for as long as 2 weeks, the dominant cell during this time being the fibroblast. Fibroblasts migrate into the wound and begin to replicate in response to mediators released during inflammation. Mediators such as C5a, fibronectin, PDGF, fibroblast growth factor (FGF), and TGF stimulate fibroblast proliferation. A cellular matrix is composed of hyaluronate and fibronectin, both of which aid in cellular migration through chemotactic factors in the wound formed during this phase of healing. Hyaluronate allows the formation of chemical gradients to attract fibroblasts. Fibronectin binds proteins and fibroblasts in a matrix and provides a pathway by which fibroblasts can move.[7] The fibroblasts bind to the arginine-glycine–aspartic acid sequence on fibronectin, a cell adhesion molecule. The fibronectin receptors on the fibroblasts then pass through the cell membrane and bind to actin filaments so that cells can migrate along the fibronectin stands according to chemotactic gradients. Fibronectin is also important in epithelialization and angiogenesis. Fibroblasts produce other proteins found in the matrix, such as proteoglycans and structural proteins. Proteoglycans are proteins to which polysaccharides can attach. Proteoglycans and hyaluronic acid are commonly found in the wound matrix. Platelet-derived growth factor is a potent stimulator of fibroblast replication and chemotaxis. Transforming growth factor β may stimulate fibroblasts to synthesize fibronectin and collagen, and EGF also stimulates collagen production.

Collagen, a family of proteins secreted by fibroblasts, is the most common protein found in the mammalian world. At least 12 types of collagen have been described. Rich in glycine and proline, collagen is formed in a tight helical structure. Cross-linking between the strands allows mature fibers to be quite resistant to breakdown. Collagen is thus an important part of mammalian structure, in addition to its role in wound healing. Macrophages control the release of collagen from fibroblasts through growth factors such as PDGF, EGF, FGF, and TGF-β. Collagen remodeling, including degradation and synthesis, may occur for up to 2 years in a healing wound. Elastin is rich in proline and lysine. In contrast to collagen, it occurs as random coils that allow some degree of stretch and recoil. It is a much less common component of wounds than collagen is.

Scar contraction occurs as the wound matures. Scar contracture may occur through the myofibroblast, a cell that is found when contraction occurs and is no longer seen after contraction is complete. However, there is still considerable debate as to the existence of the so-called myofibroblast.

Angiogenesis begins when endothelial cells begin to migrate and proliferate through a healing wound.[8, 9] New capillaries form as budding occurs from existing capillaries after stimulation by angiogenesis factors such as FGF. Transforming growth factor can also stimulate endothelial cell growth. Endothelial cells then allow connections between capillaries to form a capillary network in the healing bed. Angiogenesis is important to allow the circulation to bring new healing factors into the wound and is terminated when the wound has received an adequate blood supply. This process may be regulated by oxygen tension[10, 11]; that is, hypoxia may actually stimulate angiogenesis, and normal oxygen tensions in the wound may inhibit it.

Epithelialization occurs as cells begin to proliferate at the edge of the wound. Epithelial cells migrate over the collagen-fibronectin wound surface with the aid of contractile proteins. This process occurs until thickened mature skin covers the wound.

MATURATION

After wound repair, remodeling occurs. The scar becomes less hyperemic as the vascularity is reduced and organization and maturation of the tissues progress. Wound strength increases for up to 2 years, although the total collagen content of the wound does not increase. Thus collagen remodeling is important in wound strength. Hyaluronidase, plasminogen activators, collagenase, and elastase are involved in wound remodeling. The hyaluronate in the matrix is gradually replaced by dermatan sulfate and chondroitin sulfate, which reduce cell migration and allow cell differentiation. Plasmin formed from plasminogen degrades fibrin. Urokinase is produced by fibroblasts, endothelial cells, keratinocytes, and leukocytes and activates collagenase and elastase. Thus plasminogen activators are responsible for remodeling of the matrix and degradation of fibrin. Collagenase is secreted by macrophages, fibroblasts, epithelial cells, and white blood cells and is able to break down the collagen triple helix. Collagenase activity may be identified in the wound for many months after tissue injury.

GROWTH FACTORS

TRANSFORMING GROWTH FACTORS

Transforming growth factors are composed of two polypeptide chains.[12] They can transform the phenotype of stimulated cells and stimulate anchorage-dependent cells to lose contact inhibition and begin anchorage-independent growth. Transforming growth factor-α has amino acid homology to EGF; both bind to the FGF receptor. Transforming growth factor-β has no amino acid homology with TGF-α or any other known growth factor or protein and is quite different from TGF-α. Transforming growth factor-β is a molecule with many functions and can stimulate or inhibit the growth or differentiation of many different cells. All cells have receptors for TGF-β and can potentially respond to this growth factor. Transforming growth factor-β appears to have an important role in wound repair. It is an anabolic factor that leads to fibrosis and angiogenesis. No clinical trials have been reported on the use of TGF-α or TGF-β.

PLATELET-DERIVED GROWTH FACTOR

A polypeptide stored in the alpha-granules of platelets,[13] PDGF can also be produced by macrophages, vascular endothelium, and fibroblasts. It is composed of two chains, α and β, held together by disulfide bonds, with 60% amino acid homology between the two chains. The β-chain is quite similar to the transforming gene of the simian sarcoma virus, an acute transforming retrovirus. The human proto-oncogene C-*sis* is similar to the viral oncogene V-*sis* and codes for the β-chain of PDGF. It is a potent chemoattractant and mitogen for fibroblasts, smooth muscle cells, and inflammatory cells. It also acts with TGF-β and EGF in stimulating mesenchymal cells.[13] Although PDGF is produced by endothelial cells, endothelial cells do not respond to PDGF but work in a paracrine fashion to stimulate adjacent vascular smooth muscle cells. Smooth muscle cells also act in an autocrine fashion and produce PDGF.

Platelet-derived growth factor has been tested in several clinical trials and been shown to improve the healing of decubitus ulcers. In a trial comparing three doses of PDGF-BB homodimer, there appeared to be a benefit from PDGF in reducing the area of decubitus ulcers. Patients were treated for 28 days with PDGF at 0.01, 0.1, or 1.0 μg/cm² or with placebo.[14] Patients treated with the highest dose showed a healing response, but the lower doses had little effect. No toxicity was noted. In another study on pressure ulcers, 41 elderly patients were treated with PDGF at 100 or 300 μg/mL or with placebo for 28 days.[15] Ulcer volume was significantly reduced in the PDGF-treated groups.

A national, randomized, prospective double-blind trial comparing PDGF with vehicle alone in the treatment of 118 patients with diabetic neurotrophic foot ulcers demonstrated a significant benefit in achieving complete wound closure with PDGF.[16] Twenty-nine (48%) of 61 patients healed with PDGF, whereas only 14 (25%) of 57 patients healed with control vehicle alone. No significant adverse effects were noted with the use of PDGF.

FIBROBLAST GROWTH FACTOR

Fibroblast growth factor includes a series of heparin-bound growth factors that are potent mitogens for endothelial cells and function as angiogenesis factors by stimulating the growth of new blood vessels through the proliferation of capillary endothelial cells.[17] Two general types are acidic FGF (aFGF) and basic FGF (bFGF), with a

50% amino acid sequence homology between the two, and they interact with the same cell surface receptor. Although they are two separate entities, they both have a strong affinity for heparin. Acidic FGF is quite similar to a number of other growth factors, such as endothelial cell growth factor, whereas bFGF is similar to endothelial cell growth factor II. To date, no clinical trials have been reported on the use of aFGF or bFGF.

EPIDERMAL GROWTH FACTOR

Epidermal growth factor is a small molecule that stimulates epithelial cells. However, EGF may also stimulate fibroblasts and smooth muscle cells. Epidermal growth factor stimulates keratinocytes to grow across the wound, thus allowing wound coverage with mature skin. It has been used in clinical trials.[18] A randomized, prospective double-blind trial studied the treatment of skin graft donor sites in 12 patients to determine whether EGF would accelerate the rate of epidermal regeneration in humans. Donor sites treated with silver sulfadiazine containing EGF had an accelerated rate of epidermal regeneration as compared with paired donor sites treated with silver sulfadiazine alone. Patients treated with EGF had a shortened healing time by 1.5 days. Although these results may not have clinical significance, this study was the first prospective trial to show a benefit from a single growth factor in wound healing in humans.

In another study, EGF was used in a prospective open-label crossover trial on patients with chronic wounds.[19] Nine patients had wounds present for an average of 12 months from a variety of causes, including diabetes mellitus, rheumatoid arthritis, burn scar, or failed abdominal incision. After 3 weeks to 6 months of treatment with silver sulfadiazine without healing, the patients were crossed over to EGF at 10 μg/g of silver sulfadiazine. In eight patients, the wounds treated with EGF healed in an average of 26 to 34 days; one patient did not heal. These findings suggest that topical EGF improved wound healing.

INSULIN-LIKE GROWTH FACTOR

Insulin-like growth factors (IGFs), or somatomedins, are polypeptides that share a 50% amino acid homology with proinsulin and have insulin-like activity.[20] They circulate in an inactive state bound to a large carrier protein and appear to play a significant role in fetal growth. Somatomedin C is identical to IGF-1, whereas somatomedin is identical to IGF-2. Levels of somatomedin and IGF-1 depend on multiple factors, including the patient's age, sex, hormonal level, and nutritional status. Growth hormone is a regulator of somatomedin and IGF-1 levels, as are prolactin, thyroid hormone, and sex hormones. Elevated levels of somatomedin have been found in patients with acromegaly. They are anabolic hormones that stimulate the synthesis of glycogen, protein, and glycosaminoglycans. In addition, somatomedins stimulate the transport of glucose and amino acids across cell membranes. They can also stimulate collagen synthesis by their effect on fibroblasts. Thus far, no published clinical trials have investigated treatment with the somatomedins IGF-1 or IGF-2.

PLATELET RELEASATES

The process of wound healing is complex and involves intricate interactions between platelets and monocytes. Growth factors are initially produced by platelets in the first 48 hours after injury and thereafter by macrophages. Within the alpha-granules of platelets are a number of growth factors that are released when the platelets degranulate, including PDGF, TGF-β, FGF, platelet factor 4, EGF, β-thromboglobulin, and a platelet-derived angiogenesis factor. Preparation of a purified platelet releasate has been achieved by stimulating platelets to release the contents of their alpha-granules with thrombin.

The use of a platelet releasate has several theoretical advantages. First, the growth factors that are released are the same ones and in the same proportion as the growth factors normally released into healing wounds. Also, preparation of growth factors as a platelet releasate is relatively easy inasmuch as the platelets can be harvested from a peripheral blood sample. Because growth factors are present in banked blood, large quantities of growth factor can be gathered from pooled human blood. The major disadvantage of such a preparation, however, is the possibility of transmission of an infectious agent if the platelet releasate is used on another individual. Not all growth factors may promote healing; it is reasonable to assume the presence of some signal for wound healing to stop. Because the proper concentration of platelet releasate is unknown, a concentrated solution might not increase the effect of factors that promote wound healing but, instead, concentrate the factors that cause the wound healing process to end.

There has been considerable experience with platelet releasates in the healing of chronic wounds. A preliminary report described the use of an autologous platelet releasate in 6 patients with chronic leg ulcers secondary to connective tissue diseases and a homologous platelet releasate used in treating 11 patients with diabetic ulcers and 8 patients with venous stasis ulcers.[21] Although no benefit was observed, this study demonstrated the importance of applying topical growth factor preparations only in the context of good wound care. Growth factor preparations cannot be expected to improve wound healing unless they are applied as part of a comprehensive wound care program that also addresses the underlying wound pathology, such as venous hypertension, ischemia, or diabetic neuropathy. In another study, a series of 49 patients with chronic nonhealing cutaneous ulcers underwent treatment with autologous platelet releasate.[22] The wounds were secondary to a variety of causes, including diabetes, decubitus ulcers, venous insufficiency, arterial insufficiency, trauma, or vasculitis. The wounds had been present for an average of 198 weeks yet healed in 11 weeks after the application of autologous platelet releasate. Multivariate analysis showed a direct correlation to 100% healing with initial wound size and the initiation of platelet releasate treatment. This was the first clinical series to demonstrate that a combination of locally acting growth factors promote the healing of chronic ulcers.

In a randomized prospective trial of platelet releasate vs. a platelet buffer as placebo, both were added to microcrystalline collagen and then applied to wounds secondary to diabetes, peripheral vascular disease, venous stasis, or vasculitis.[23] Thirty-two patients were randomized and then treated for 8 weeks. In the group receiving platelet releasate, 81% of the patients had epithelialization at 8 weeks as compared with 15% in the control group. After crossover to treatment with platelet releasate, patients in the control group had epithelialization in an average of 7 weeks. This study, then, showed a significant effect of topically applied growth factors. It must be noted, however, that the growth factors were added to microcrystalline collagen, which is a potent stimulator of platelets, and the contribution of the collagen to the healing was not defined.

A homologous platelet releasate was used to treat intractable ulcers.[24] Twenty-three patients received standard wound care without evidence of healing for an average period of 25 weeks. Then after a control period of 3 months during which they were treated with saline and silver sulfadiazine, the patients were treated with topical silver sulfadiazine and a homologous preparation of platelet releasate. During the control period, three ulcers healed. However, treatment with homologous platelet releasate healed all the remaining ulcers. For diabetic neurotrophic ulcers, the average time to healing was 7 weeks. For venous stasis ulcers, the average time to healing was 14 weeks. Age, sex, location of the ulcer, and ulcer duration had no influence on the probability of healing.

In a randomized, prospective double-blind study of 70 patients with diabetic neurotrophic foot ulcers, platelet releasate or placebo was applied topically to the ulcer. During the 20-week trial, 80% of the patients achieved complete wound healing with a platelet releasate, whereas only 29% healed with saline placebo. All patients in this study had adequate arterial blood flow in the wound, were free of infection, and had extensive débridement of the wounds before entry.[25]

Another trial observed very different results with a homologous platelet releasate.[26] In a randomized, prospective, double-blind placebo-controlled trial, topical platelet releasate was applied to leg ulcers in 26 patients. The ulcers were caused by diabetes mellitus, peripheral vascular disease, or venous disease and had been present for an average of 5 months. Wounds treated with platelet releasate increased in size, whereas wounds in the control group improved, i.e., became smaller. This study suggested no benefit of platelet releasate over standard care in treating lower extremity ulcers.

Thirteen patients with diabetic neurotrophic ulcers were entered into a randomized, prospective double-blind trial of platelet releasate vs. saline placebo.[27] A statistically significant benefit in treating these ulcers with platelet releasate was noted. After 20 weeks of treatment, 5 of 7 patients treated with platelet releasate had healed, whereas only 2 of 6 patients treated with saline control had healed. By 24 weeks, another 3 of the 6 patients in the control group had healed, which suggests that the platelet releasate stimulated more rapid healing but perhaps did not result in a greater proportion of wound healing.

Although the results of clinical trials using platelet releasates have been varied, the bulk of the data suggests that there is a beneficial effect to using platelet releasate in the treatment of chronic ulcers of the lower extremity. Indeed, this group of growth factors may ultimately play a significant role in the adjunctive treatment of ischemic ulcers.

HYPERBARIC OXYGEN

Wound healing is significantly decreased by a hypoxic environment. Hypoxia can cause lowered levels of fibroblast proliferation, collagen production, and capillary angiogenesis.[28, 29] Oxygen-dependent leukocyte bacterial killing of the aerobic organisms found in wound infections is also impaired, thus creating the ideal environment in which anaerobic and microaerophilic organisms flourish. Hyperbaric oxygen (HBO) can restore a favorable cellular milieu in which the wound healing process and host antibacterial mechanisms are enhanced.[30]

A substantial portion of HBO therapy is based on its ability to halt the associated infective process in most wounds. A reduction in oxygen tension below 30 mm Hg significantly impairs bacterial killing by polymorphonuclear leukocytes.[31] Hence, by simply elevating the effective tissue oxygen tensions, antimicrobial therapy may be enhanced. In addition, the increased oxygen tensions have a direct lethal effect on anaerobic organisms.

Hyperbaric oxygen therapy can also provide an increase in tissue oxygenation of hypoperfused wound. This elevation in oxygen tension directly promotes wound healing by enhancing fibroblast replication, collagen synthesis, and neovascularization. Evidence also suggests that HBO may prepare an ischemic vascular bed for skin grafting.

Before HBO therapy is initiated on any open skin wound, identification of the underlying etiology and risk factors that may inhibit tissue healing is crucial. Effective management requires noninvasive vascular studies and accurate transcutaneous oximetry determinations (tissue oximetric readings near the ulcer that are consistently less than 30 mm Hg in a nonedematous extremity). Thus, a trial of adjunctive therapy with HBO at 2.0 and 2.5 atm for 90 to 120 minutes may be tried in problem ischemic wounds if arterial insufficiency has been appropriately treated.[32, 33] It should be emphasized, however, that HBO therapy is not a substitute for arterial revascularization; rather, it should be considered for ischemic wounds only in situations in which revascularization and/or operative débridement have failed to positively alter the healing process.

CONCLUSION AND SUMMARY OF GROWTH FACTORS

Growth factors applied topically to wounds can acclerate wound healing by stimulating granulation tissue formation and enhancing epithelialization. Transforming growth factors, although isolated in various stages of wound healing, have yet to be tested in clinical trials. Platelet-derived growth factor has been shown to be effective in decubitus (pressure) ulcers and diabetic neurotrophic ulcers. Fibroblast growth factor has been shown to increase angiogenesis in ex vivo experiments, but to date no significant clinical trials have been performed to demonstrate this effect on human wounds. Epidermal growth factor stimulates epithelial cells, and clinical trials have shown that it aids in epidermal regeneration in skin graft donor sites and in chronic nonhealing wounds. Insulin-

TABLE 2.

Summary of Clinical Trials and Current Availability of Growth Factors

Growth Factor	Clinical Trials (References)	Availability
TGF	Ongoing	NA
PDGF	14–16	NA
FGF	None	NA
EGF	18, 19	NA
IGF	None	NA
Platelet releasates	21–27	Procuran (Curative Health Services)
HBO	32, 33	Widely available

Abbreviations: TGF, transforming growth factor; *PDGF,* platelet-derived growth factor. *FGF,* fibroblast growth factor; *EGF,* epidermal growth factor; *IGF,* insulin-like growth factor; *HBO,* hyperbaric oxygen.

like growth factor appears to stimulate collagen synthesis and the transport of glucose and amino acids across cell membranes. However, like FGF, no clinical trials have demonstrated its efficacy in wounds. The most promising results thus far stem from clinical trials using platelet releasates containing a combination of growth factors. These trials have demonstrated efficacy in the healing of a variety of wounds, including pressure, diabetic, venous, and ischemic ulcers.

In conclusion, although the results of studies in venous, pressure, and diabetic ulcers appear to be promising, the role of topical growth factors in the treatment of arterial insufficiency–related ischemic ulcers is not yet clearly defined (Table 2). New investigations using combinations of HBO therapy and growth factors in conjunction with lower extremity revascularization are needed. Finally, we emphasize the critical role of adequate débridement as an important adjunct to any clinical application of growth factors and/or HBO therapy.[34] It is clear at this stage, however, that topical growth factor or HBO therapy should be not considered a substitute for appropriate surgical débridement or revascularization.

REFERENCES

1. Hunt TK, LaVan EB: Enhancement of wound healing by growth factors. *N Engl J Med* 321:111–112, 1989.

2. McGrath MH: Peptide growth factors and wound healing. *Clin Plast Surg* 17:421–432, 1990.

3. Rothe MJ, Falanga V: Growth factors and wound healing: *Clin Dermatol* 9:553–559, 1992.

4. Edington HE: Wound healing, in Simmons RL, Steed DL (eds): *Basic Science Review for Surgeons.* Philadelphia, WB Saunders, 1992, pp 41–55.

5. Steed DL: Mediators of inflammation, in Simmons RL, Steed DL (eds): *Basic Science Review for Surgeons.* Philadelphia, WB Saunders, 1992, pp 12–29.

6. Steed DL: Hemostasis and coagulation, in Simmons RL, Steed DL (eds): *Basic Science Review for Surgeons.* Philadelphia, WB Saunders, 1992, pp 30–37.

7. Grinnel F: Fibronectin and wound healing. *Am J Dermatopathol* 4:185–192, 1982.

8. Folkman T, Klansburn M: Angiogenic factors. *Science* 235:442–447, 1987.

9. Pevec WC, Ndoye A, Brinsky JL, et al: New blood vessels can be induced to invade ischemic skeletal muscle. *J Vasc Surg* 24:534–544, 1996.

10. Knighton DR, Hunt TK, Schewenstuhl A: Oxygen tension regulates the expression of angiogenesis factor by macrophages. *Science* 221:1283–1290, 1983.

11. Knighton DR, Silver IA, Hunt TK: Regulation of wound healing angiogenesis: Effect of oxygen gradients and inspired oxygen concentration. *Surgery* 90:262–269, 1981.

12. Sporn MB, Roberts AB: Transforming growth factor. *JAMA* 262:938–941, 1989.

13. Lynch SE, Nixon JC: Role of platelet-derived growth factor in wound healing: Synergistic effects with growth factors. *Proc Natl Acad Sci U S A* 84:7696–7697, 1987.

14. Robson M, Phillips L: Platelet-derived growth factor BB for the treatment of chronic pressure ulcers. *Lancet* 339:23–25, 1992.

15. Mustoe T, Cutler N: A phase II study to evaluate recombinant platelet-derived growth factor-BB in the treatment of stage 3 and 4 pressure ulcers. *Arch Surg* 129:212–219, 1994.

16. Steed DL, Diabetic Ulcer Study Group: Clinical evaluation of recombinant human platelet-derived growth factor for the treatment of lower extremity diabetic ulcers. *J Vasc Surg* 21:71–81, 1995.

17. Folkman J, Klagsburn M: Angiogenic factors. *Science* 235:442–447, 1987.

18. Brown GL, Nanney LB: Enhancement of wound healing by topical treatment with epidermal growth factor. *N Engl J Med* 321:76–80, 1989.

19. Brown GL, Curtsinger L: Stimulation of healing of chronic wounds by epidermal growth factor. *Plast Reconstr Surg* 88:189–194, 1991.

20. Spencer EM, Skover G, Hunt TK: Somatomedins: Do they play a pivotal role in wound healing? In Barbul A, Pines E, Caldwell M (eds): *Growth Factors and Other Aspects of Wound Healing: Biological and Clinical Implications.* New York, Alan R Liss, 1988.

21. Steed DL, Goslen B, Hambley R, et al: Clinical trials with purified platelet releasate, in Barbul A (ed): *Clinical and Experimental Approaches to Dermal and Epidermal Repair: Normal and Chronic Wounds.* New York, Alan R Liss, 1990, pp 103–113.

22. Knighton DR, Ciresi KF: Classifications and treatment of chronic nonhealing wounds. *Ann Surg* 104:322–330, 1986.

23. Knighton DR, Ciresi K: Stimulation of repair in chronic, nonhealing, cutaneous ulcers using platelet-derived wound healing formula. *Surg Gynecol Obstet* 170:56–60, 1990.

24. Atri SC, Misra J: Use of homologous platelet factors in achieving total healing of recalcitrant skin ulcers. *Surgery* 108:508–512, 1990.

25. Holloway GA, Steed DL, DeMarco MJ, et al: A randomized controlled dose response trial of activated platelet supernatant topical CT-102 (APST) in chronic nonhealing wounds in patients with diabetes mellitus. *Wounds* 5:198–206, 1993.

26. Krupski WC, Reilly LM: A prospective randomized trial of autologous platelet-derived wound healing factors for treatment of chronic nonhealing wounds: A preliminary report. *J Vasc Surg* 14:526–532, 1991.

27. Steed DL, Goslen JZB, Holloway GA, et al: CT-102 activated platelet supernatant, topical versus placebo: A randomized prospective double blind trial in healing of chronic diabetic foot ulcers. *Diabetes Care* 15:1598–1604, 1992.

28. Ehrlich HP, Grislis G, Hunt TK: Metabolic and circulatory contributions to oxygen gradients in wounds. *Surgery* 72:578–583, 1972.

29. La Van FB, Hunt TK: Oxygen and wound healing. *Clin Plast Surg* 17:463–472, 1990.

30. Ninikoski J, Hunt TK, Zederfeldt B: Oxygen supply in healing tissue. *Am J Surg* 123:247–252, 1972.

31. Beauman L, Beauman BL: The role of oxygen and its derivatives in microbial pathogenesis and host defense. *Annu Rev Microbiol* 38:27–48, 1984.

32. Wattel F, Mathieu D, Coget JM, et al: Hyperbaric oxygen therapy in chronic vascular wound management. *Angiology* 41:59–65, 1990.

33. Roth RN, Weiss LD: Hyperbaric oxygen and wound healing. *Clin Dermatol* 12:141–156, 1994.

34. Steed DL, Donohoe D, Webster MW: Effect of extensive debridement and treatment on the healing of diabetic foot ulcers. *J Am Coll Surg* 183:61–64, 1996.

Index

A

Abciximab, 217
Abdominal aortic aneurysms (*see also* Thoracoabdominal aortic aneurysm resection)
  critical pathways for, 83–92
    discussion, 89–91
    patients and methods, 84–88
    results, 88
  laparoscopic aortic surgery for, 147–148
  spiral computed tomography in repair of, 115–131
    accessory renal arteries and inferior mesenteric artery patency and, 126–127
    anatomic features in planning of repair and, 119–120
    associated structures and, 127–129
    clinical considerations, 119
    extent of aneurysm and, 120–122
    occlusive disease of aortic branches and, 122–126
    technical considerations, 116–119
Ablative atherectomy, 175
Adamkiewicz, artery of, 98–99, 101
Amputation, in Raynaud's syndrome, 53, 54, 55, 58
Anastomotic aneurysms, in hemodialysis access site failure, 74
Anatomy
  of brachiocephalic arteries, pathologic, 27–28, 29–30
  of spinal cord blood supply, 96–99
Ancrod, 218–219
Anesthesia
  in endovascular treatment of brachiocephalic lesions, 12–13
  in hemodialysis access, 66–67

Aneurysms
  abdominal aortic (*see* Abdominal aortic aneurysms)
  anastomotic, in hemodialysis access site failure, 74
  mycotic (*see* Mycotic aneurysms)
  subclavian artery, 58
  ulnar artery, 57–58
Angiogenesis, in wound healing, 228–229
Angiography
  of abdominal aortic aneurysms, 115
  in atherectomy, 181–183
  failing dialysis grafts and, 79
  magnetic resonance, in brachiocephalic disease, 31
  of mycotic aneurysms, 163, 164
  in renal artery diseas, 189–190
  in upper extremity ischemia, 49–52, 56, 57
Angioplasty
  atherectomy vs., 176
  in brachiocephalic vessels, 11–12, 18
    access and equipment, 13
    clinical experience, 21–22
    complications, 20
  failing dialysis grafts and, 79
Anterior cerebral ischemia, 30–31
Anterior spinal artery, 97–98
Antibiotics, in mycotic aneurysms, 166
Antibodies, heparin and, 204, 207–208
Anticardiolipin antibodies, heparin and, 204
Anticoagulants, 201–221
  agents available, 201
  coumarin derivatives
    complications, 213–214
    initiating warfarin therapy, 210
    monitoring warfarin therapy, 211–212

239

G

Gas embolism, in laparoscopic aortic
surgery, 142
Glycoprotein IIB/IIIA inhibitors,
217
Grafts
for abdominal aortic aneurysms,
147–148
aortobifemoral bypass, laparoscopy
and, 134–135, 140–141, 143,
144–147
in brachiocephalic arterial
reconstruction, 34–35,
36–37
in hemodialysis, 62–63, 68–71
infection of, 73–74
seromas and, 74–75
in mycotic aneurysms, 167, 168,
169
Great radiculomedullary artery,
98–99, 101
Growth factors, in wound healing,
223–238
clinical trials and current
availability, 236
epidermal growth factor, 224, 231,
235, 236
fibroblast growth factor, 224,
230–231, 235, 236
fibroplasia and, 227, 228
insulin-like growth factor, 224,
231–232, 235–236
platelet-derived growth factor, 224,
228, 230, 235, 236
platelet releasates, 232–234
transforming growth factors, 224,
228, 229–230, 235, 236

H

Helical computed tomography (*see*
Spiral computed tomography)
Hemasite, 63
Hematomas, puncture site, in
hemodialysis access site
failure, 75

Hemodialysis
central venous catheters for, 71–72
goal of perfect access site in,
61–63
procedures for access, 61
Hemodialysis access site failure,
61–82
anesthesia issues in, 66–67
causes, 72
choice of new sites in, 70–71
coagulation issues in, 65–66
definition and nature of, 63–65
general approaches to, 65
nonsurgical treatment of failing
site, 79–80
special issues
access site problems, 73
anastomotic aneurysms, 74
carpal tunnel syndrome, 78
edema, 78–79
errors by dialysis personnel, 76
errors in site selection, 75–76
graft infection, 73–74
ischemia and vascular steal,
77–78
patient-related problems, 76–77
puncture site hematomas, 75
seromas, 74–75
strategy of long-term hemodialysis
access and, 63
surgical revision in, 67–70
Hemorrhage, warfarin and, 213–214
Hemostasis, hemodialysis access
and, 69–70
Heparin and heparin-like
anticoagulants
administration and monitoring,
204–205
complications, 206–208
in endovascular treatment of
brachiocephalic lesions, 20
hemodialysis and, 66
heparinoids, 202, 203, 207
low molecular weight heparin,
202, 203, 205, 206, 207–208
pharmacokinetics, 203